Other monographs in the series, Major Problems in Clinical Surgery:

Child: *The Liver and Portal Hypertension*

Welch: *Polypoid Lesions of the Gastrointestinal Tract*

Madding and Kennedy: *Trauma to the Liver*

Barker: *Peripheral Arterial Disease*

Spratt and Donegan: *Cancer of the Breast*

Haller: *Deep Thrombophlebitis*

Colcock and Braasch: *Surgery of the Small Intestine in the Adult*

Jackman and Beahrs: *Tumor of the Large Bowel*

Ellis and Olsen: *Achalasia of the Esophagus*

Botsford and Wilson: *The Acute Abdomen*

Colcock: *Diverticulitis*

Spratt, Butcher and Bricker: *Exenterative Surgery of the Pelvis*

Shires: *Shock*

Child: *Portal Hypertension*

In Collaboration With

CORNELIUS E. SEDGWICK, M.D.
HORST S. FILTZER, M.D.
WILLIAM A. MEISSNER, M.D.
HENRY E. ZELLMAN, M.D.
FERRIS J. SIBER, M.D.
GEORGE O. BELL, M.D.
BENTLEY P. COLCOCK, M.D.
JOHN R. BOOKWALTER, M.D.
MORRIS J. NICHOLSON, M.D.
JOSEPH P. CREHAN, M.D.

SURGERY OF THE THYROID GLAND

by

Cornelius E. Sedgwick, M.D.

Surgeon, Lahey Clinic Foundation; Chairman, Department
of Surgery, New England Deaconess Hospital; Surgeon,
New England Baptist Hospital, Boston, Massachusetts

Volume XV in the Series
MAJOR PROBLEMS IN CLINICAL SURGERY

J. ENGLEBERT DUNPHY, M.D.
Consulting Editor

W. B. Saunders Company   Philadelphia, London, Toronto   1974

W. B. Saunders Company: West Washington Square
Philadelphia, PA 19105

12 Dyott Street
London, WC1A 1DB

833 Oxford Street
Toronto, Ontario M8Z 5T9, Canada

Library of Congress Cataloging in Publication Data

Sedgwick, Cornelius E

Surgery of the thyroid gland.

(Major problems in clinical surgery, v. 15)

1. Thyroid gland–Surgery.   I. Title.   [DNLM: 1. Thyroid gland–Surgery.   W1 MA492R v. 15 1974 / WK280 S448s]

RD599.S42   617'.5395   73-80981

ISBN 0-7216-8048-8

Surgery of the Thyroid Gland   ISBN 0-7216-8048-8

© 1974 by W. B. Saunders Company. Copyright under the International Copyright Union. All rights reserved. This book is protected by copyright. No part of it may be reproduced, stored in a retrieval system, or transmitted in any form or by any means, electronic, mechanical, photocopying, recording, or otherwise, without written permission from the publisher. Made in the United States of America. Press of W. B. Saunders Company. Library of Congress catalog card number 73-80981.

Last digit is the Print No.:   9   8   7   6   5   4   3   2   1

Foreword

In this volume Dr. Cornelius Sedgwick and his colleagues present a remarkably complete, up-to-date documentation of all aspects of the surgery of the thyroid gland, from basic anatomy and physiology to the finer details of technical surgery, anesthesia and patient care.

The chapters on thyroid physiology by Dr. Zellman and thyroid isotopology by Dr. Siber are an exceptionally valuable reference source for clinicians and surgeons not primarily engaged in work in these areas.

Dr. Sedgwick recommends a logical and appropriately conservative approach to the surgery of thyroid cancer and supports his position with extensive references from the literature.

The chapter on surgical technique is a gem—well worth the price of the book for residents seeking competence in this precise and exacting surgical field.

In short, this is a splendid addition to the series on major problems in clinical surgery. It should have wide appeal to residents, practicing surgeons and academicians.

J. Englebert Dunphy

Preface

This book is written for students, clinicians, and surgeons interested in thyroid disease. Great advances have been made in the last decade in thyroidology, which has become an accepted subspecialty of medicine. Few surgeons can keep abreast of the advances in endocrinology and biochemistry of the thyroid gland. Yet those surgeons who operate on the thyroid gland must have a basic knowledge of anatomy, pathology, and physiology of the normal thyroid as well as of changes caused by disease states as we understand them today.

The surgeon must appreciate other methods and modalities of treating thyroid disease. The patient with altered thyroid function or tumor is best treated by group consultation of internists, thyroidologists, pathologists, isotopologists, and therapeutic radiologists. Diagnosis and treatment may involve one or more of these modalities. If surgery is decided upon, the surgeon must be able to excise the proper amount of thyroid tissue, with morbidity and mortality approaching zero.

The purpose of this book is to help those interested in thyroid surgery to have a ready reference to the anatomy, pathology, and physiology of the thyroid gland, the diagnosis and treatment of thyroid disease, and, lastly, the therapeutic armamentarium available for treating thyroid disease. The authors of these chapters have worked together for more than a quarter of a century and have seen almost all thyroid patients before they are operated on. The toxic or hyperthyroid patients have all been brought into a euthyroid state by Dr. George O. Bell and Dr. Henry E. Zellmann. The removed specimens have all been studied by members of the same Laboratory of Pathology at the New England Deaconess Hospital, which was first directed by Dr. Shields Warren and later by Dr. William A. Meissner. The anesthesia has been given by the same technique described by Dr. Morris J. Nicholson, and the surgical procedures have been performed by a relatively small group of surgeons using essentially the same technique first described by Dr. Frank H. Lahey. We believe this is the ideal way of treating thyroid disease. The reader will learn how each member of our "thyroid team" plays his part in the care of the patient with thyroid disease. I wish to acknowledge their willingness to contribute chapters to this book.

I am grateful, also, for the editorial work of Charlotte R. Thompson, Pauline A. Zorolow, and the staff of the Editorial Department of the Lahey Clinic Foundation, for the excellent illustrations and drawings prepared by P. D. Malone and Francis E. Steckel of the Art Department of the Lahey Clinic, for the photography of George L. Buchanan of the Photographic Department of the Lahey Clinic, and, lastly, to the W. B. Saunders Company for not only publishing the book but for the patience and kindly probing which brought the book to its conclusion.

CORNELIUS E. SEDGWICK, M.D.

Contents

Chapter One

    OPERATIVE HISTORY OF GOITER 1
    Cornelius E. Sedgwick, M.D., and Horst S. Filtzer, M.D.

Chapter Two

    EMBRYOLOGY AND DEVELOPMENTAL ABNORMALITIES 5
    Cornelius E. Sedgwick, M.D.

Chapter Three

    SURGICAL ANATOMY 10
    Cornelius E. Sedgwick, M.D.

Chapter Four

    SURGICAL PATHOLOGY 24
    William A. Meissner, M.D.

Chapter Five

    THYROID PHYSIOLOGY AND FUNCTIONAL TESTS 55
    Henry E. Zellmann, M.D.

Chapter Six

    THE SURGICAL SIGNIFICANCE OF THYROID ISOTOPOLOGY:
    MORPHOLOGIC AND PHYSIOLOGIC CONSIDERATIONS 71
    Ferris J. Siber, M.D.

Chapter Seven

    HYPERTHYROIDISM 99
    George O. Bell, M.D.

Chapter Eight

> NONTOXIC NODULAR GOITER (ADENOMATOUS GOITER) 121
> *Cornelius E. Sedgwick, M.D.*

Chapter Nine

> THYROIDITIS 126
> *Bentley P. Colcock, M.D.*

Chapter Ten

> THYROID TUMORS 133
> *Cornelius E. Sedgwick, M.D., and John R. Bookwalter, M.D.*

Chapter Eleven

> ANESTHESIA FOR THYROID SURGERY 153
> *Morris J. Nicholson, M.D., and Joseph P. Crehan, M.D.*

Chapter Twelve

> SURGICAL TECHNIQUE 170
> *Cornelius E. Sedgwick, M.D.*

INDEX 203

Chapter One

OPERATIVE HISTORY OF GOITER

Cornelius E. Sedgwick, M. D.
and
Horst S. Filtzer, M.D.

"Thus, whether we view this operation in relation to the difficulties which must necessarily attend its execution, or with reference to the severity of the subsequent inflammation, it is equally deserving of rebuke and condemnation. No honest and sensible surgeon, it seems to me, would ever engage in it."[7]

From the historical information available, it is not entirely clear when surgery and goiter met. Ancient authors often did not distinguish between scrofula and goiter; therefore, a precise date is not possible. Paulus,[20] of Aegina, is believed by some to have performed the first extirpation for goiter around the year 500 A.D. Albucasis,[1] of Baghdad, the prolific writer of 30 books on medicine and surgery, is credited as being the first to perform successful excision of goiter around the year 1,000 A.D. Being a "bold and venturesome operator," he is said to have rescued a patient from the hands of a homo ignarus who had a great deal of trouble controlling hemorrhage from the thyroid gland. Skillfully using both ligature and cautery, Albucasis successfully controlled the bleeding, and, apparently, performed several successful extirpations for goiter himself.

Until 1363 when Guy de Chauliac[5] reaffirmed the feasibility of surgery for goiter, superstition and fear surrounded the thyroid gland; treatment for goiter had consisted of the application of toad blood, the stroking of the gland with a cadaver's hand, and other bizarre remedies. De Vigo,[6] in his literature written from 1501 to 1512, described several extirpations for goiter, as did Lusitanus[14] in 1550, but the surgical approach to goiter remained shrouded by disbelief and superstition.

Muys,[19] in 1629, described ligature of the thyroid arteries as a method of treating goiter in animals. Von Walther[23] subsequently described in detail the surgical approach to the treatment of goiter by ligature of the superior thyroid arteries. Several reports appear in the mid-eighteenth century of successful extirpation for the treatment of large goiters, including several successful reports from von Langenbeck's clinic.

Mandt[17] in 1832 reported his own successful case of excision of a large goiter and gave an extensive review of the literature up to that time. His operation, which took one hour, was remarkable in that the specimen weighed 18 ounces. No anesthesia was available at that time; the ultimate result was quite successful, although the patient fainted on three occasions during the operation.

In 1864 Günther[8] tabulated all surgical procedures performed up to that time, and Bruberger[3] in 1876 tabulated 124 cases, with an operative mortality of 29 percent. Surprisingly, Günther's cases were not included in Bruberger's report, but he clearly stated in his paper the indications for thyroidectomy and recommended it as the procedure of choice for the alleviation of respiratory distress resulting from large goiters.

By the end of the nineteenth century, thyroidectomy had become an acceptable form of surgical therapy. Billroth[2] had performed 20 operations with eight operative deaths by 1883. It is clear that these were total extirpations of the gland, as tetany was a major cause of the resulting deaths. Weiss[24] reported in 1883 that tetany resulted after total thyroidectomy, but the significance of the parathyroid glands was not appreciated until the work of von Eiselsberg,[22] a pupil of Billroth's, showed that removal of these glands alone resulted in tetany. MacCallum and Voegtlin[15] in 1909 showed that control of calcium was mediated by the parathyroid glands, thus more clearly defining the relationship. The reader is referred to the excellent work of Halsted[9] in 1924 for a review of the entire operative story of goiter.

The greatest single contributor to the field of thyroid surgery is Theodor Kocher.[12] As early as 1878 he reported 13 consecutive thyroidectomies with only two deaths. Born in Bern, Switzerland, in 1841, he was a student of Billroth's and, subsequently, professor of surgery at Bern from 1877 until his death in 1917. This man, without a doubt, was the greatest contributor to the field of thyroid surgery. By 1912 he had performed more than 5,000 thyroidectomies; with the care and gentleness he exercised, successful operations were almost a foregone conclusion. When he noted that "cachexia strumipriva," or myxedema, developed in a number of his initial patients, his painstaking research led him to advocate subtotal thyroidectomy as the procedure of choice.

Although thyroxin was not isolated until 1915 by Kendall,[11] thyroid surgery was becoming accepted practice with most of the major clinics in this country which specialized in the field. The work of Plummer[21] in 1923, using Lugol's iodine solution to suppress the toxic gland before operation, deserves a great deal of credit, but the world of surgery owes its greatest gratitude to Kocher, who, in 1909, received the Nobel prize in medicine for his work.

The operative history of goiter cannot be complete without mentioning the names of those American individuals who set thyroid surgery well on its way toward becoming the most effective method for the treatment of goiter, be it Graves' disease, toxic goiter, or nontoxic goiter.

William Stewart Halsted,[10] returning from his studies in Europe, began thyroid surgery at The Johns Hopkins University by performing transplantations of the thyroid glands in dogs. In 1888 he developed clamps to control bleeding and showed that a perfectly dry operative field was necessary to permit the surgeon to operate efficiently in an orderly procedure. He advocated thyroidectomy for Graves' disease and wrote the first chapter on thyroid surgery in the United States.

The Mayo brothers[18] in Rochester, Minnesota, were introduced to surgery of the thyroid in 1890 when they operated on a huge goiter in a healthy, 60-year-old Scotsman. Hemorrhage from the lesion was controlled by ligation and by packing with turpentine-soaked sponges. The patient did well, and the interest in thyroid surgery by the Mayo brothers continued. In 1904 Charles Mayo received an honorary master of arts degree from Northwestern University. In a paper presented to the American Surgical Association he pointed out that in 40 cases of Graves' disease, thyroidectomy successfully treated the disease. Although initially the mortality rates were high, by 1912 Charles Mayo, with persistent work and improvements in technique, had operated on 278 patients with exophthalmic goiter without a death. He emphasized precise technique and division of the strap muscles to improve exposure and to prevent tetany by preserving the parathyroid glands by meticulous dissection.

Crile[4] developed a meticulous technique for allaying the fear and anxiety of preoperative patients with Graves' disease in order to prevent thyroid storm after operation. He believed that anxiety precipitated the thyroid storm, and that if the surgeon could "steal" the gland without the patient's knowing about it, anxiety would be prevented. To do this, he gradually introduced the patient to an "inhalation treatment" and then, without the patient's actual knowledge, he proceeded with the surgical therapy. It was said that some of his patients were discharged from the hospital without ever knowing that a portion of the thyroid gland had been removed. By 1932, because of his exacting technique and "safe" surgery, he and his associates had carried out some 22,000 operations on the thyroid gland, nearly half of which had been for the relief of thyrotoxicosis, with a mortality of 1 percent.

Similarly, Frank Lahey,[13] while a house officer at Boston City Hospital, became interested in surgery of the thyroid gland and was the first surgeon to use the basal metabolic test as an index of hyperthyroidism. Long before the era of antithyroid drugs and with the use of iodine and the judicious use of a two-stage or three-stage procedure, he was able to lower the mortality rate of subtotal thyroidectomy for Graves' disease to less than 1 percent. This was a remarkable achievement, for many of the patients came to operation with basal metabolic rates of 75 to 100. Like many of his predecessors, Lahey had to fight the prejudices of his medical colleagues, and in 1918, at the age of 38, he published an article reporting the 190 operations which he had performed for the treatment of goiter. This article showed the striking results that could be obtained by surgery. Throughout his career Lahey and his colleagues operated on more than 18,000 patients with thyroid problems, and more than 5,000 of those operations were for Graves' disease. The operative mortality rate was 0.7 percent. The technique of "safe" surgery which he taught is still practiced at the Lahey Clinic today.

In the beginning of the 1940's MacKenzie and Astwood,[16] working on the development of antithyroid drugs, were able to produce propylthiouracil, which somewhat changed the treatment of Graves' disease. As the active gland was now much more amenable to control, it made thyroid surgery infinitely safer. Little more need be said about the recent advent of radioiodine therapy, improvement in the antithyroid drugs, and radioisotope scanning techniques; they are all now well established modalities.

It remains, however, that surgery for goiter continues to be a superb method of therapy which, in skilled hands, is safe and curative.

REFERENCES

1. Albucasis: Quoted by Mandt: Der Kropf: Geschichte und Exstirpation desselben. Rust's Magazin fur die gesammte Heilkunde 37:387, 1832.
2. Billroth: Quoted by Halsted.
3. Bruberger: Ueber die Exstirpation des Kropfes, nebst einem geheilten Fall von Totalexstirpation einer grossen, mit breiter Basis aufsitzenden Struma hyperplastica und statistischen Bemerkungen. Deutsch. Militär. Z. 5:176, 1876.
4. Crile: Quoted by Colcock, B. P.: Lest we forget: A story of five surgeons. Surgery 64:1162–1172 (Dec.) 1968.
5. de Chauliac, G.: Quoted by Halsted.
6. de Vigo: Quoted by Günther.
7. Gross, S. D.: A System of Surgery. 4th ed. Philadelphia, Lea & Febiger, 1866, p. 394.
8. Günther: Quoted by Halsted.
9. Halsted, W. S.: The operative story of goitre. The author's operation. Johns Hopkins Hosp. Rep. 19:71–257, 1920.
10. Halsted: Quoted by Colcock.
11. Kendall: Quoted by Major, R. H.: A History of Medicine. Vol. 2. Springfield, Illinois, Charles C Thomas, 1954, pp. 926–927, 998, 1001.
12. Kocher: Quoted by Klebs, A. C.: Theodor Kocher 1841–1917. U.S. Naval Med. Bull. 12:59–63 (Jan.) 1918.
13. Lahey: Quoted by Colcock.
14. Lusitanus: Quoted by Halsted.
15. MacCallum and Voegtlin: Quoted by Major.
16. MacKenzie and Astwood: Quoted by Means, J. H., DeGroot, L. J., and Stanbury, J. B.: The Thyroid and Its Diseases. 3rd ed. New York, McGraw-Hill Book Co., 1963.
17. Mandt: Quoted by Halsted.
18. Mayo brothers: Quoted by Colcock.
19. Muys: Quoted by Garrison, F. H.: An Introduction to the History of Medicine. 4th ed. Philadelphia, W. B. Saunders Company, 1929.
20. Paulus: Quoted by Halsted.
21. Plummer: Quoted by Major.
22. von Eiselsberg: Quoted by Major.
23. von Walther: Quoted by Garrison.
24. Weiss: Quoted by Halsted.

Chapter Two

EMBRYOLOGY AND DEVELOPMENTAL ABNORMALITIES

Cornelius E. Sedgwick, M.D.

It is essential that the thyroid surgeon be familiar with the embryology of the thyroid gland so that he will appreciate the possible developmental abnormalities that may occur as well as the various possible locations for ectopic thyroid tissue. The thyroid takes its origin from epithelium in the midline of the floor of the pharynx, which forms the median thyroid diverticulum. The diverticulum increases in size and shape and grows downward as a hollow stalk, the thyroglossal duct. As the median thyroid diverticulum descends in the midline at the level of the thyroid cartilage, it grows laterally into the lateral lobes of the thyroid. The thyroglossal duct may persist or differentiate into thyroid tissue at any level. Its distal end may become the pyramidal lobe. Normally the epithelium of the thyroglossal duct undergoes degeneration and atrophy and disappears. Occasionally the epithelium remains, and at any site along the duct, cysts, fistulas, or ectopic thyroid tissue may develop (Fig. 2-1).

THYROGLOSSAL CYSTS AND FISTULAS

Thyroglossal cysts and fistulas may occur anywhere between the base of the tongue and the suprasternal notch. They are essentially near the midline structures, more often on the left than on the right side. They occur at the foramen caecum linguae, above or below the hyoid, in the area of the thyroid gland, or in the region of the suprasternal notch. Occasionally the thyroglossal duct above the cyst will remain patent. Pressure on such a cyst may express fluid into the mouth at the foramen caecum.

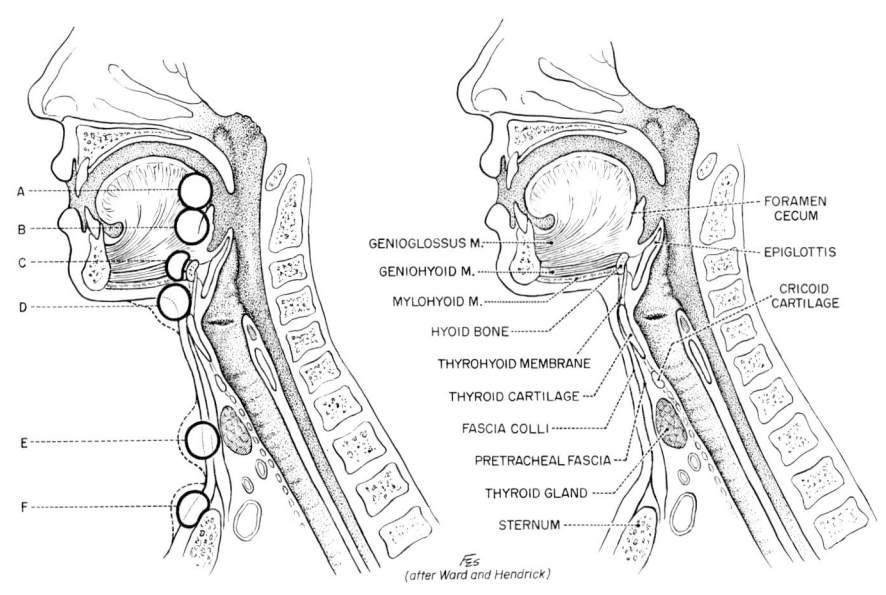

Figure 2–1. Location of thyroglossal cysts. A, In front of foramen cecum; B, at foramen cecum; C, suprahyoid; D, infrahyoid; E, area of thyroid gland; and F, suprasternal.

Thyroglossal cysts are prone to infection; they may drain spontaneously or require incision. Infection of the cyst frequently is the reason patients seek medical attention. Drainage of an infected cyst leads to formation of a thyroglossal fistula. A fistula may close spontaneously and repeated drainage may be necessary. Noninfected cysts should be excised, never drained. Noninfected cysts, other than those located at the base of the tongue, produce few symptoms. Thyroglossal cysts at the base of the tongue may cause mild dysphasia. A thyroglossal cyst below the hyoid may be mistaken for an adenoma of the pyramidal lobe. An adenoma elevates with swallowing, a thyroglossal cyst does not; a thyroglossal cyst elevates with protrusion of the tongue, an adenoma does not.

The treatment of thyroglossal cysts and fistulas is surgical excision. The entire cyst and thyroglossal duct must be removed up to the foramen caecum. The duct may pass anterior or posterior to the hyoid bone or through the bone. To prevent recurrence, the midsection of the hyoid should be excised, as advocated by Sistrunk.[5]

ECTOPIC THYROID

Defects in the developmental descent of the thyroglossal duct may result in abnormal location of thyroid tissue. Failure of or incomplete descent gives rise to midline ectopic thyroid rests. The commonest is the pyramidal lobe, extending upward from the isthmus or from either lateral lobe. The pyramidal lobe is important to the thyroid surgeon treating Graves' disease. It may be small, overlooked, and responsible for recurrent hyperthyroidism. The less common median thyroid rest is lingual thyroid located at the base of the tongue (Fig. 2–2). Although lingual thyroid usually is the only functioning thyroid tissue, normally situated thyroid may also be present.[1,3] Symptoms of lingual goiter depend upon its size. Its growth may be secondary to physiologic hypertrophy or tumor. The patient may be aware of interim oral swelling. As it becomes large it may produce dysphasia, dyspnea, and dysphonia. Diagnosis of lingual thyroid may be confirmed by ^{131}I scan (Fig. 2–3). If malignant disease is suspected, a biopsy should be taken. As lingual goiter may be the only functioning thyroid tissue, a trial of thyroid extract for suppression or iodine-131 for shrinkage is indicated. Lingual goiter should be excised only if it is producing symptoms. Excision may produce myxedema, in which case permanent thyroid replacement therapy must be instituted.

Other sites of median thyroid rests as remnants of the thyroglossal duct are below or above the hyoid. Such supra- or infrahyoid goiters, as in lingual thyroid, may be the only functioning thyroid tissue. They appear as discrete masses, are usually asymptomatic, and may be mistaken for thyroglossal cysts. Iodine-131 scan and biopsy are necessary for diag-

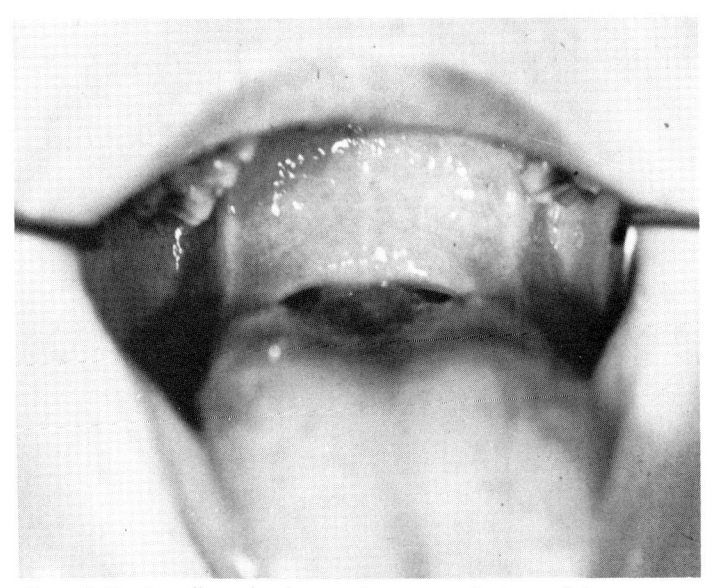

Figure 2–2. Intralingual goiter can be seen at the base of the tongue.

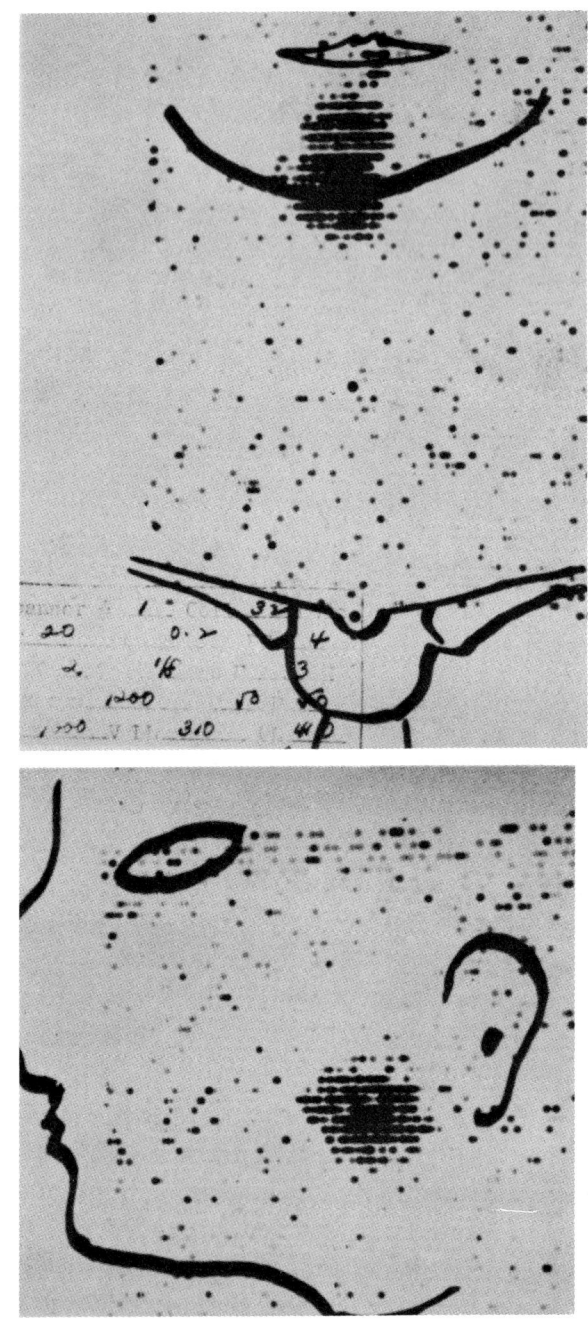

Figure 2–3. Thyroid scan of a 4-year-old girl showing lingual location of the thyroid. Top, front view; bottom, side view. (From Rogers, W. M.: Normal and anomalous development. *In* Werner, S. C., and Ingbar, S. H. (eds.): The Thyroid: A Fundamental and Clinical Text. 3rd ed. New York, Harper & Row, 1971.)

nosis. As in a normally placed goiter, carcinoma may arise in median ectopic thyroid. Excellent reviews may be found in the literature.[2, 4]

On rare occasions ectopic thyroid tissue has been found in the periaortic region, the pericardium, the heart, and the diaphragm. Such developmental thyroid rests are the result of the displacement of thyroid remnants into the mediastinum by the heart as it migrates downward over the primitive thyroid.[5]

REFERENCES

1. Buckman, L. T.: Lingual thyroid. Laryngoscope 46:765–784; 878–897; 935–955 (Oct., Nov., Dec.)
2. Fish, J., and Moore, R. M.: Ectopic thyroid tissue and ectopic thyroid carcinoma: A review of the literature and report of a case. Ann. Surg. 157:212–222 (Feb.) 1963.
3. Montgomery, M. L.: Lingual thyroid. A comprehensive review. West. J. Surg. 43:661–669 (Dec.) 1935.
4. Shepard, G. H., and Rosenfeld, L.: Carcinoma of thyroglossal duct remnants. Review of the literature and addition of two cases. Amer. J. Surg. 116:125–129 (July) 1968.
5. Sistrunk, W. E.: Surgical treatment of cysts of thyroglossal tract. Ann. Surg. 71:121–123 (Feb.) 1920.

Chapter Three

SURGICAL ANATOMY

Cornelius E. Sedgwick, M.D.

Surgeons attempting operations on the thyroid gland must be well informed on the anatomy of the neck, including the thyroid gland, its blood supply and its nerve supply, as well as its adjacent structures—the trachea, larynx, and esophagus, and the parathyroids. The gross anatomy of the thyroid gland is described elsewhere (Chapter 4). This chapter deals with the surgical anatomy of the thyroid as it applies to surgical procedures discussed elsewhere in this book. It is presented in a topographical manner, describing the anatomy as it is encountered in thyroidectomy.

THE SKIN

The skin of the neck may reveal several transverse folds which may be of value in deciding the site of an incision. A group of folds may occur just above the sternum and clavicle, and one such fold may be ideal for a low collar incision.

THE MUSCLES

The *platysma* is a thin, sheet-like muscle immediately beneath the skin in the subcutaneous area, spreading in a fan-like fashion from below the clavicle laterally to the mandibles above, leaving a space in the midline (Fig. 3–1). When the skin flaps are turned up to expose the underlying muscles, the skin, subcutaneous fat, and platysma should be dissected as a single layer. By this means, unnecessary bleeding will be avoided, since the fascial plane between the platysma and the fascia covering the prethyroid muscles is quite avascular.

The muscles which must be dealt with during thyroid surgery are

SURGICAL ANATOMY

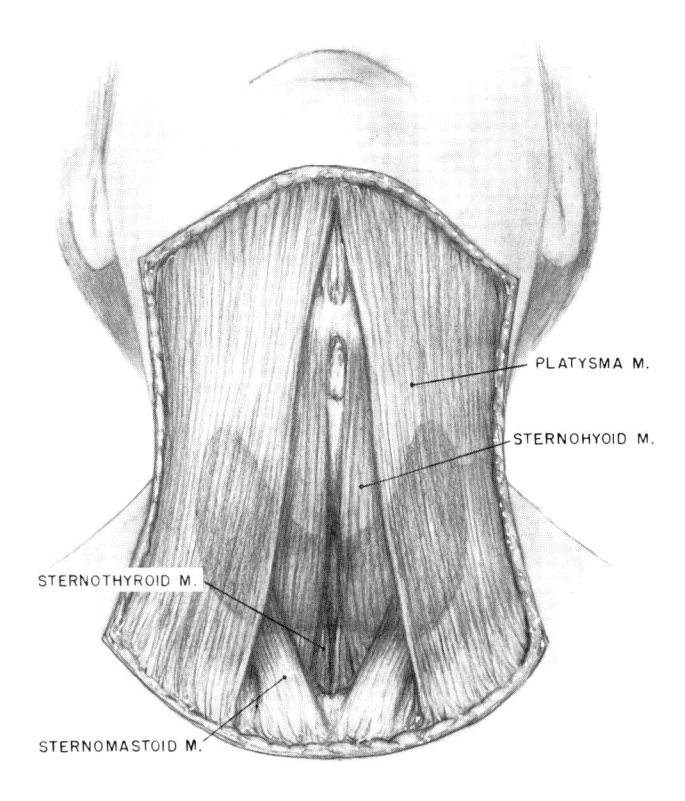

Figure 3-1. Fan-like spread of platysma from mandibles to clavicles. The sternohyoid and sternothyroid muscles are seen in midline. The platysma fibers are best visualized for excision at lateral margins.

the two lateral *sternocleidomastoid* muscles, forming the lateral boundaries, and the *sternohyoid* and *sternothyroid* muscles, forming the superficial and anterior boundaries (Fig. 3-2). Both the sternohyoid, lying more anterior, and the sternothyroid, just beneath and covering the thyroid capsule, arise from the sternum. The sternohyoid attaches above to the hyoid, and the sternothyroid attaches to the thyroid cartilage. The fascia of the anterior medial border of the sternocleidomastoid fuses with the fascia of the lateral border of the sternohyoid. This is divided longitudinally during exposure of the thyroid to allow retraction of the sternocleidomastoid laterally and the sternohyoid medially. The nerve supply to the sternohyoid and sternothyroid is the ansa hypoglossi. This nerve descends along the lateral border of the sternohyoid and enters the muscles low in the neck. If the sternohyoid and sternothyroid are to be divided transversely, they must be transected high to preserve the motor function of this nerve.

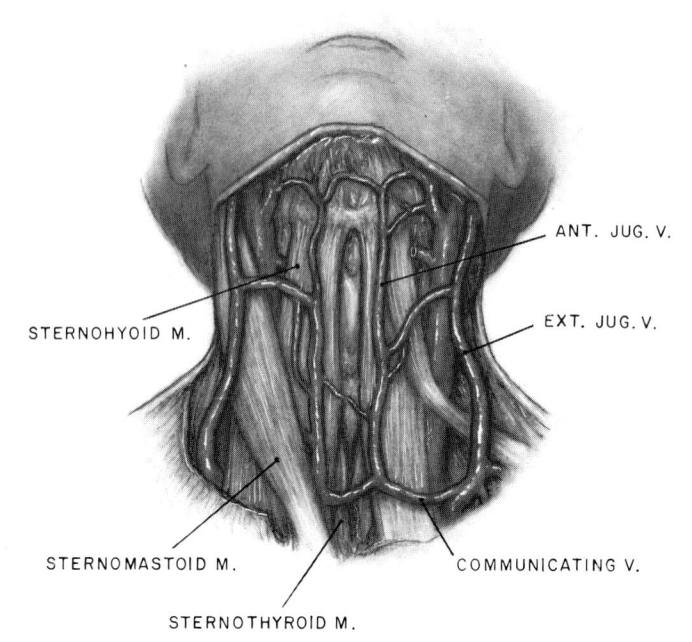

Figure 3-2. Right side, The muscles. Lateral, The sternocleidomastoid muscle passes upward from the sternoclavicular joint to the mastoid process. Medial, The sternohyoid passes from the sternum to the hyoid. The sternothyroid, posterior to the sternohyoid, is visualized low in the neck close to its attachment to the sternum.

Left side, The superficial veins. The sternocleidomastoid muscle has been removed. Note communicating veins between the external and anterior jugular veins.

THE BLOOD VESSELS

The principal blood vessels to and from the thyroid gland are external to the capsule and can be ligated before the gland is entered. The superior and inferior thyroid arteries constitute the main arterial supply. Occasionally a branch from the aorta or innominate artery, the thyroidea ima artery, and the thyroidea ima vein enter from below. The veins, in general, drain to the corresponding arteries.

THE VEINS

The *superficial veins* lie beneath the platysma (Fig. 3-2). They are easily visualized and should present no problem for the thyroid surgeon. The external jugular veins are lateral and cross over the belly of the sternocleidomastoid. The anterior jugular veins immediately overlie the sternohyoid muscles. A plexus of communicating veins may be present between the external and anterior jugular veins. In large goiters the superficial veins may be of considerable size. Care should be exercised in turning up the skin flaps with the platysma so that the veins are not cut.

Surgical Anatomy

If the surgeon carefully divides the fascia between the sternocleidomastoid and the sternohyoid, the communicating veins may be ligated and divided. The external jugular vein may then be retracted laterally along with the sternocleidomastoid. The anterior jugular vein is divided when the sternohyoid and sternothyroid are transected.

The *deep thyroid veins* leave the gland in relationship to the thyroid arteries mainly at the superior and inferior poles and the lateral aspect of the gland (Fig. 3-3). They are less constant than the arteries in number, position, and size. The deep veins may be a serious threat during thyroid surgery because they are numerous and may easily be torn, with ensuing hemorrhage. This is particularly true in large, substernal goiters. In such cases the clavicle may act as a tourniquet and produce great dilatation and increased pressure in the veins. If uncontrolled hemorrhage occurs, the lower pole and the substernal extension of the goiter must be quickly mobilized out of the mediastinum. Release of the tourniquet effect of the clavicle will allow the veins to collapse and the hemorrhage will be brought under control

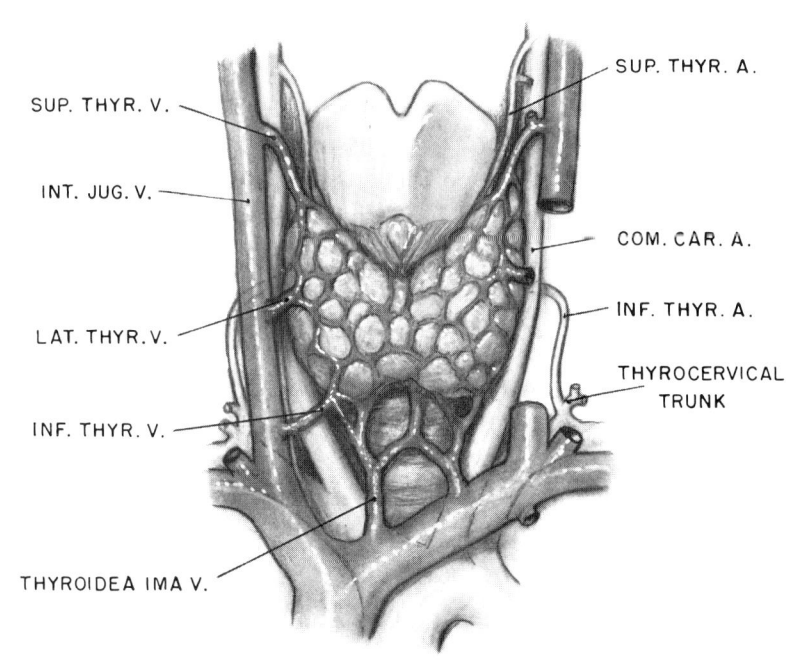

Figure 3-3. Right, The deep veins drain into the internal jugular veins. The superior thyroid vein is lateral to the superior thyroid arteries. The lateral or medial thyroid veins may vary in number from one to four. The inferior thyroid veins may form a plexus emptying into the internal jugular vein or present as the thyroidea ima vein emptying into the innominate vein.

Left, The arteries. The superior thyroid artery, a branch of the external carotid artery, gives off a branch to the pyramidal lobe and isthmus. The inferior thyroid artery arises from the thyrocervical trunk, passes upward posterior to the carotid sheath, and then loops downward into the midsection of the gland.

The *superior thyroid vein* leaves the gland at the superior pole just anterior and lateral to the superior thyroid artery. It empties into the cricothyroid tributary of the internal jugular vein. It is ligated along with the superior thyroid artery during thyroidectomy.

The *lateral* or *middle* veins vary greatly in number. They pass directly from the lateral border of the lobes and enter into the internal jugular vein. During thyroidectomy they must be divided to allow access to the lateral compartment. In pathologically enlarged glands, the jugular vein and the lateral thyroid veins may be pushed close to the capsule of the thyroid. In such cases they may be mistaken for veins in the thyroid capsule, and the fascial plane between the thyroid and the jugular vein may be difficult to find. The lateral veins may override the capsule and must be identified and divided before an attempt is made to enucleate the gland.

The *inferior thyroid vein* leaves the lower pole in one or more trunks, frequently forming a plexus of veins. The inferior thyroid vein is not adjacent to the inferior thyroid artery, which is in the region of the middle third of the gland. The inferior thyroid artery is more closely associated with the lateral thyroid vein. The inferior thyroid vein empties into the internal jugular vein and occasionally directly into the innominate vein. Occasionally a thyroidea ima vein drains the isthmus, passing downward on the trachea to enter the left innominate vein. The inferior thyroid veins may be closely interwoven with the recurrent nerve as it ascends. This is a vulnerable area for injury to the recurrent laryngeal nerve.

The Arteries

Superior Thyroid Artery

The superior thyroid artery arises as the first branch from the external carotid artery at about the level of the bifurcation of the common carotid artery (Fig. 3-3). It runs downward and medially on the surface of the inferior constrictor muscles, entering the upper pole of the thyroid on its anterior-superior surface. In its downward course it is just inferior and lateral to the superior laryngeal nerve. The superior laryngeal nerve usually turns medial from the superior thyroid artery about 1 cm. above the pole. Care, then, must be exercised in ligating the superior thyroid artery close to its entrance to the gland to avoid injury to the superior laryngeal nerve. In many pathologically enlarged thyroid glands there is a lingula of thyroid tissue above and lateral to the point of entry of the superior thyroid artery and the superior laryngeal nerve. If this lingula is mistaken for the upper pole, the artery may be ligated too high with possible damage to the superior laryngeal nerve. Occasionally a branch of the superior thyroid artery to the pyramidal lobe and isthmus may arise high, and bleeding may occur from the upper pole after ligation of the superior thyroid artery simply because the artery was ligated below the origin of this branch to the pyramidal lobe.

Inferior Thyroid Artery

The inferior thyroid arteries arise from the thyrocervical trunks shortly after their origin from the subclavian arteries. They ascend upward behind the jugular veins and carotid arteries to a level above the inferior pole of the thyroid. Then they make a loop downward and medially and enter the gland at its midportion, not at the inferior pole as frequently stated in some texts. The surgeon's first glimpse of the inferior thyroid artery is usually when the thyroid gland is retracted medially and the jugular vein laterally. It appears from beneath the carotid artery opposite the midsection of the thyroid. Before entering the thyroid the inferior thyroid artery may divide into one or more branches and be intimately associated with one or more branches of the superior laryngeal nerve. (See description of nerve.) One branch of the inferior thyroid artery may supply the inferior parathyroid. Great care must be used in ligating the inferior thyroid artery in this region to avoid injury to the recurrent laryngeal nerve. It should not be ligated until the recurrent nerve and its branches are visualized, and then it should be ligated as far laterally as possible.

The *thyroidea ima artery* may be present, although this is unusual in my experience. It arises from the aorta or innominate artery and passes directly upward in front of the trachea to enter the lower border of the isthmus. It is usually ligated with the inferior thyroid veins.

THE LYMPHATIC SYSTEM

Knowledge of the lymphatic vessels draining the thyroid is essential in planning radical surgical procedures. In general, the lymphatics accompany the veins. Collecting lymph channels draining the intraglandular capillaries are found beneath the thyroid capsule. These channels drain into the lymph vessels associated with the capsule and may cross-communicate with the isthmus and opposite lobe, the direction of flow being toward the right (Figs. 3-4 and 3-5).

The *superior lymph vessels* drain the isthmus and the medial superior portion of the thyroid lobes, ascending in front of the larynx and terminating in the subdigastric lymph nodes of the internal jugular chain.

The *median inferior lymph vessels* descend with the inferior vein to the pretracheal nodes. The *lateral collecting group*, above, follows the superior thyroid vessels to the anterior and superior nodes of the internal jugular chain and, below, follows the lateral thyroid and inferior thyroid veins to the lateral and inferior nodes of the internal jugular vein. These internal jugular pretracheal and anterior jugular nodes can usually be excised surgically by a radical neck dissection. Tumor invading the pretracheal nodes, however, may spread downward into the anterior-superior me-

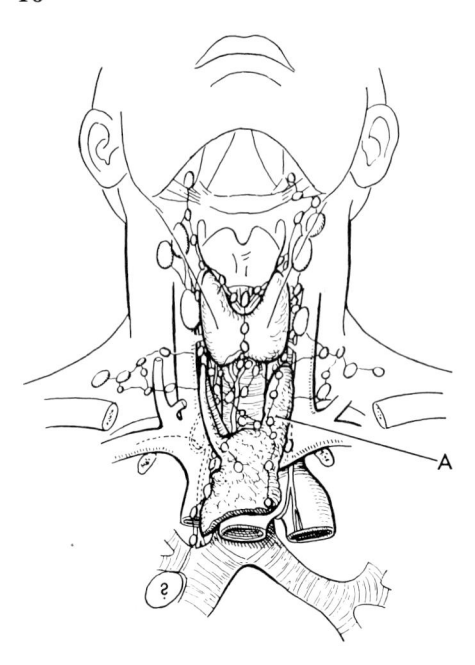

Figure 3–4. Lymphatics. Distribution of the lymphatics from the thyroid in the more superficial planes. A, Thymus; its upper poles in the neck lie medial to the internal jugular vein. (Adapted from Werner, S. C., and Ingbar, S. H. (eds.): The Thyroid, a Fundamental and Clinical Text. New York, Harper & Row, 1971.)

Figure 3–5. Lymphatics. Areolar spaces around the thyroid containing local (B, C, D) and regional (E, F, G) lymphatics from the gland. A, Corner of gland after superior pole has been mobilized and drawn forward, showing relationship of corner to entrance of a branching recurrent laryngeal nerve. The right side is shown on the figure because the preponderance of spread of cancer in the thorax is to the right even though the primary disease may be in the lower part of the left lobe or isthmus. (Adapted from Werner, S.C., and Ingbar, S.H. (eds.): The Thyroid, a Fundamental and Clinical Text. New York, Harper & Row, 1971.)

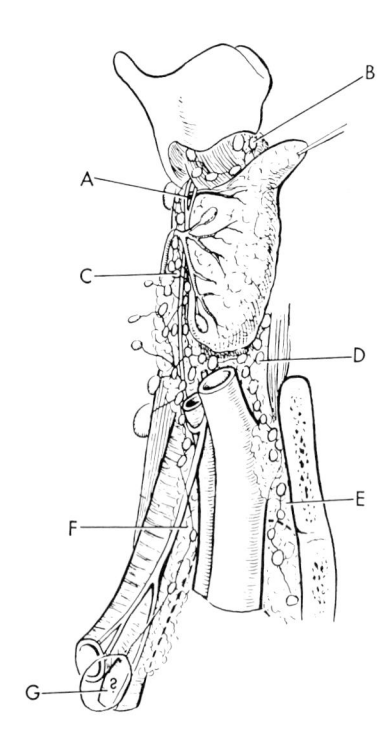

SURGICAL ANATOMY

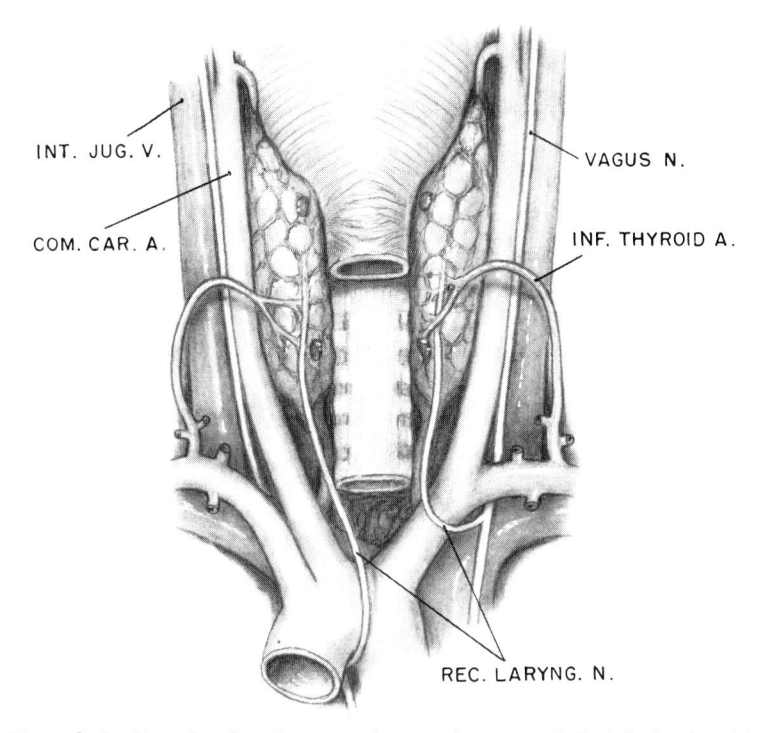

Figure 3-6. Posterior view. Recurrent laryngeal nerves and the inferior thyroid arteries. The recurrent laryngeal nerves as they ascend in the region of the lower pole of the thyroid are lateral to the tracheal groove.

diastinal nodes out of reach of the usual radical neck dissection. McClintock[7] advises that in selected cases, if the pretracheal nodes and the anterior mediastinal nodes are involved with differentiated tumor, a transsternal dissection of the anterior mediastinum should be combined with the usual radical neck dissection.

Another group of lymphatics draining the posterior-superior aspect of the thyroid leaves the posterior capsule and passes to the retropharyngeal nodes. Rouvière[11] found this to be present in one fifth of his dissections. Obviously, if the retropharyngeal nodes are involved in tumor, they are not eradicated by a radical neck dissection.[7, 11]

THE NERVES

The *recurrent laryngeal nerves* arise from the vagus at different levels on the two sides (Fig. 3–6). The right recurrent laryngeal nerve arises where the vagus crosses the first portion of the subclavian artery. The nerve hooks around the lower and posterior aspect of the subclavian artery and ascends lateral to the trachea, entering the larynx posterior to the thyroid at the cricothyroid articulation. The left recurrent laryngeal nerve leaves the vagus as the vagus crosses over the arch of the aorta; it hooks around the aorta and ascends again as the right recurrent nerve does, lateral to the trachea to its terminal branches within the laryngeal muscles.

As emphasized by Fowler and Hanson,[4] the usual textbook description of the nerves descending in the groove between the rounded surfaces of the trachea and esophagus at the lower pole of the thyroid out of harm's way was not found in their dissection of 400 recurrent nerves. They stated, and this has been our experience, that the nerves in the region of the lower pole of the thyroid gland are 1 to 2 cm. lateral to the trachea. At this level, as the recurrent laryngeal nerve ascends to the middle third of the thyroid gland, it may consist of extralaryngeal branches closely associated with the inferior thyroid artery. It may pass posterior or superficial to the inferior thyroid artery, or its extralaryngeal branches may intertwine in innumerable variations. Rarely does the recurrent laryngeal nerve branch below the inferior thyroid artery. Therefore, it is safer to search for the nerve below the artery. This is the most vulnerable area for injury to the recurrent laryngeal nerve. Reed[9] lists 28 types of relationships of the recurrent laryngeal nerve to the inferior thyroid artery (Fig. 3-7). Recent investigation by Dedo[3] indicates that the recurrent laryngeal nerve has only one motor trunk innervating the laryngeal muscles (Fig. 3-8). The other extralaryngeal branches are sensory, one of which may join the sensory branch of the superior laryngeal nerve to form the loop of Galen (Fig 3-8).

From the practical point of view the thyroid surgeon must consider each extralaryngeal branch of the recurrent nerve as the possible motor nerve supplying the laryngeal muscles and make every attempt at preserving them all. At the posterior-lateral aspect of the thyroid capsule, the recurrent laryngeal nerve appears to penetrate and pass through the thyroid gland. It continues upward and medially in close relationship with the posterior capsule of the middle third of the thyroid gland and enters the larynx between the arch of the cricoid cartilage and the inferior cornu of the thyroid cartilage. Whether the nerve actually enters the gland substance or is merely in very close apposition to the capsule is of no great importance to the thyroid surgeon if, when mobilizing the posterior aspects of the gland, he is aware of this close relationship.

The recurrent nerve, on rare occasions, does not recur. It may pass directly across from the vagus beneath the inferior constrictor fibers in close apposition to the superior thyroid vessels to the larynx (Fig. 3-9). It is for this reason that we identify the recurrent laryngeal nerve before the superior thyroid vessels are ligated.

The *superior laryngeal nerve* arises from the vagus close to the base of the skull, descends medially to the carotid vessels and, at the level of the hyoid cornu, divides into two branches. The internal branch is sensory;

Surgical Anatomy

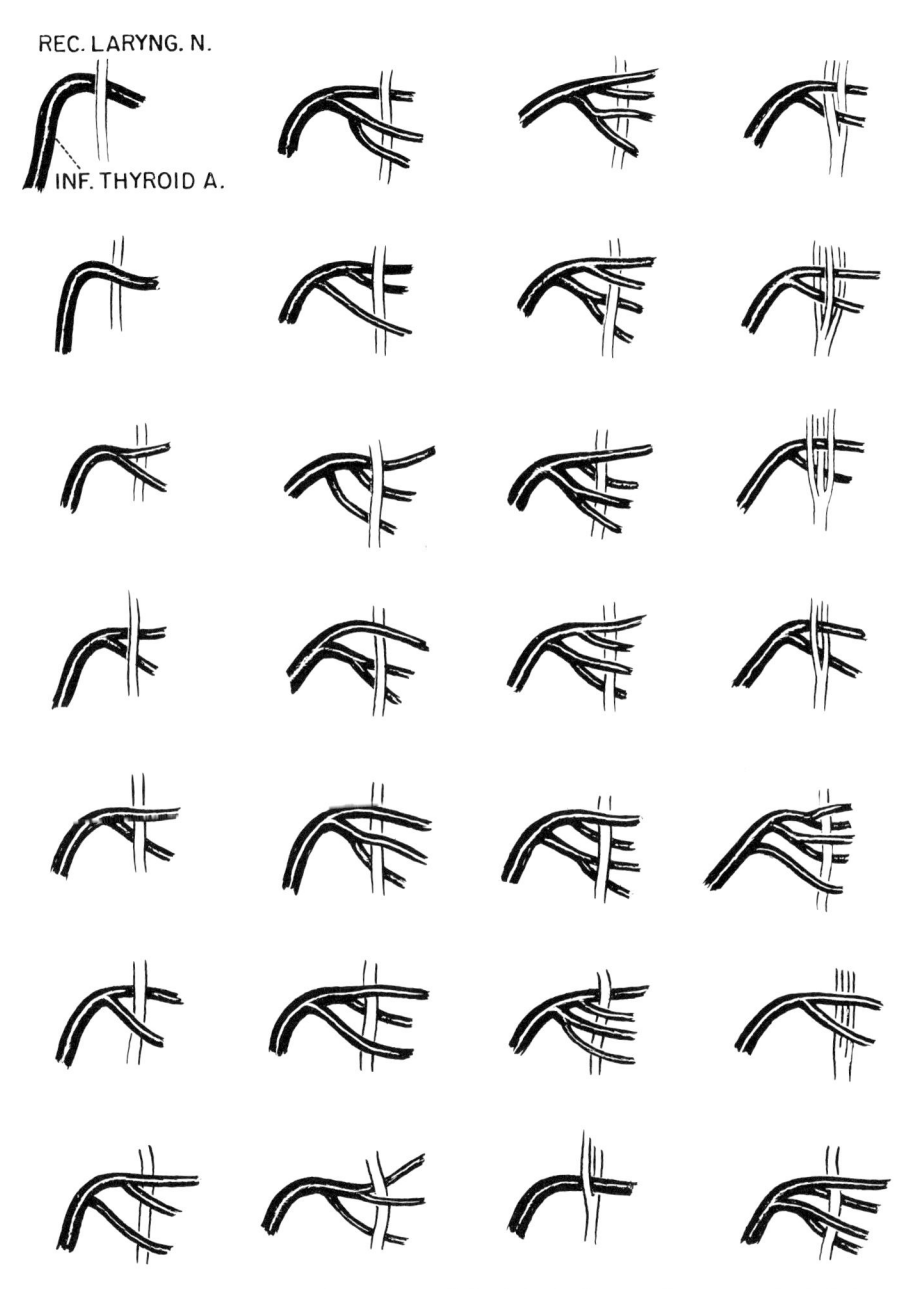

Figure 3-7. Types of relationships of the inferior laryngeal nerve to the inferior thyroid artery. (Adapted from Reed, A. F.: Anat. Rec. 85:18, 1943.)

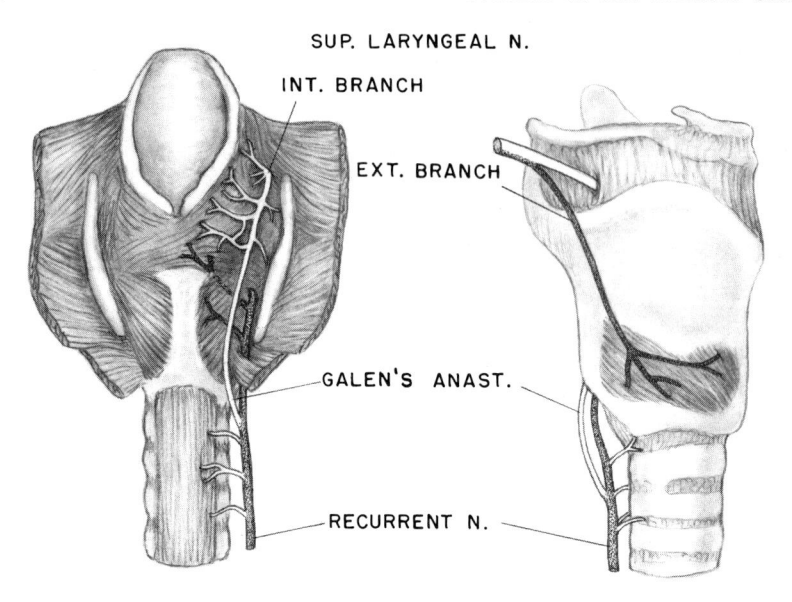

Figure 3-8. Recurrent laryngeal nerve has only one motor branch to the laryngeal muscles. The other extralaryngeal branches are sensory, one of which joins the sensory branch of the superior laryngeal nerve to form the loop of Galen. Superior laryngeal nerve divides into two branches: the internal or motor branch innervates the cricothyroid muscle, and the lateral or sensory branch forms the loop of Galen. (Adapted from Dedo, H.H.: Laryngoscope 80:1467, 1970.)

it penetrates the thyrohyoid membrane and may anastomose with the sensory branch of the recurrent laryngeal nerve to complete the loop of Galen (Fig 3-8). The external branch of the superior laryngeal nerve lies on the lateral surface of the inferior pharyngeal constrictor muscle and descends to innervate the cricothyroid muscle. Both branches lie immediately adjacent to the superior thyroid artery and may be injured if the superior thyroid artery is ligated "in bulk" too high above its entrance into the thyroid gland.

If the recurrent nerve is injured, paralysis of the vocal cord occurs on the ipsilateral side. Controversy exists concerning an explanation for the position of the paralyzed cord and the neuromuscular mechanism involved. The laryngeal muscles, five on each side, involving motion of the vocal cords, are the abductors (the internal arytenoid and the thyroarytenoid), and the adductors (the lateral posterior cricoarytenoid), and are innervated by the recurrent laryngeal nerve. The cricothyroid muscle, which has to do with range of voice (the tensors of the vocal cord), is innervated by the internal branch of the superior laryngeal nerve. Early investigators, particularly Rosenbach[10] (1880) and Semon[13] (1881), postulated that the abductor fibers of the recurrent nerve are more susceptible to pressure than the adductor fibers—the

Surgical Anatomy

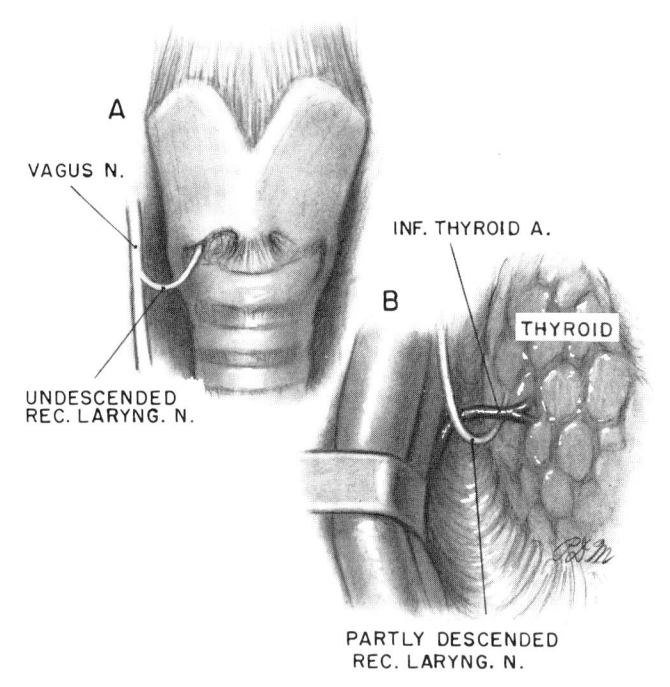

Figure 3-9. *A*, The unusual but occasional undescended inferior laryngeal nerve passing directly from vagus to beneath the horn of the thyroid cartilage (nonrecurrent laryngeal nerve). *B*, Partly descended recurrent nerve passing underneath the inferior thyroid artery but not descending into the chest.

Semon-Rosenbach Law. Wagner[14] (1890) and Grossmann[5] (1897) stated that paralysis of the vocal cord in the paramedian position was the result of injury of the recurrent laryngeal nerve and that paralysis of the cord in the intermediate position was the result of injury of the recurrent laryngeal nerve and the superior laryngeal nerve—the Wagner-Grossmann theory. Another popular theory was based on the extralaryngeal branchings of the recurrent nerves.[1, 2, 6, 8, 12, 15] This hypothesis assumed that the extralaryngeal branches went to abductors or adductors. Division of the adductor branch would place the cords in an abducted position, and injury to the abductor fibers would place the cord in an adductor position.

Dedo,[3] in an excellent paper, reviewed the many theories on the innervation of the larynx and the mechanism of laryngeal paralysis (Fig. 3-9). He also studied laryngeal paralysis in dogs and human beings, correlating clinical and electromyographic findings, and concluded that the "behavior of paralyzed vocal cords is best explained by the Wagner-Grossmann theory—that complete paralysis of the recurrent nerve causes a vocal cord to be immobilized in the paramedian position, and combined paralysis of the recurrent laryngeal and superior laryngeal

INSPIRATION   PHONATION

NORMAL

PARAMEDIAN

INTERMEDIATE

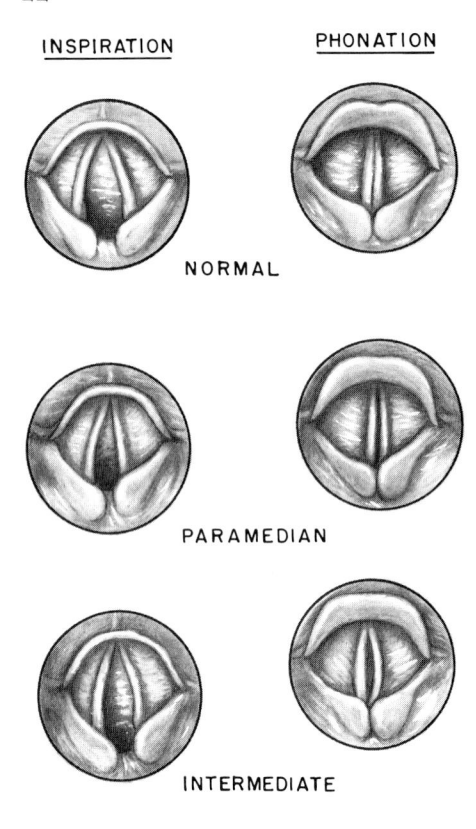

Figure 3-10. Human vocal cord shape and position during inspiration and phonation caused by specific laryngeal nerve paralyses. Normal, recording position of electrodes in intrinsic muscles; paramedian, right recurrent nerve paralysis; intermediate, right recurrent and superior laryngeal nerve paralysis. Note the medial prominence of vocal process seen best during inspiration. (Adapted from Dedo, H. H.: Laryngoscope 80:1470, 1970.)

nerves causes a vocal cord to be paralyzed in the intermediate position" (Fig. 3-10). Furthermore, he found no evidence to support the concept of extralaryngeal branching into abductor and adductor trunks.

REFERENCES

1. Armstrong, W. G., and Hinton, J. W.: Multiple divisions of recurrent laryngeal nerve; anatomic study. Arch. Surg. 62:532-539 (April) 1951.
2. Berlin, D. D., and Lahey, F. H.: Dissections of recurrent and superior laryngeal nerves; relation of recurrent to inferior thyroid artery and relation of superior to abductor paralysis. Surg. Gynec. Obstet. 49:102-104 (July) 1929.
3. Dedo, H. H.: The paralyzed larynx: An electromyographic study in dogs and humans. Laryngoscope 80:1455-1517 (Oct.) 1970.
4. Fowler, C. H., and Hanson, W. A.: Surgical anatomy of thyroid gland with special reference to relations of recurrent laryngeal nerve. Surg. Gynec. Obstet. 49:59-65 (July) 1929.
5. Grossmann, M.: Experimentelle Beiträge zur Lehre von der Posticuslähmung. Arch. Laryngol. Rhinol. 6:282-360, 1897.
6. King, B. T., and Gregg, R. L.: Anatomical reason for the various behaviors of paralyzed vocal cords. Ann. Otol. 57:925-944 (Dec.) 1948.
7. McClintock, J. C.: Thyroid cancer: Choice of surgical procedure. *In* Young, S., and Inman, D. R.: Thyroid Neoplasia. Symposium on Thyroid Neoplasia, London, 1967. New York, Academic Press, 1968, pp. 80-102.

8. Morrison, L. F.: Recurrent laryngeal nerve paralysis; revised conception based on dissection of 100 cadavers. Ann. Otol. 61:567–592 (June) 1952.
9. Reed, A. F.: Relations of inferior laryngeal nerve to inferior thyroid artery. Anat. Rec. 85:17–23 (Jan.) 1943.
10. Rosenbach, O.: Zur Lehre von der doppelseitigen totalen Lähmung des Nerv laryngeus inferior (recurrens). Breslau Aerztl. Z. 2:14–16; 27–30 (Jan. and Feb.) 1880.
11. Rouvière, H.: Anatomy of the Human Lymphatic System. A compendium translated from the original "Anatomie des Lymphatiques de l'Homme" and rearranged for the use of students and practitioners by M. J. Tobias. Ann Arbor, Michigan, Edward Brothers, 1938.
12. Rustad, W. H.: Revised anatomy of recurrent laryngeal nerves: Surgical importance, based on dissection of 100 cadavers. J. Clin. Endocr. 14:87–96 (Jan.) 1954.
13. Semon, F.: Clinical remarks on the proclivity of the abductor fibres of the recurrent laryngeal nerve to become affected sooner than the adductor fibres, or even exclusively, in cases of undoubted central or peripheral injury or disease of the roots or trunks of the pneumo-gastric, spinal accessory, or recurrent nerves. Arch. Laryngol. Rhinol. 2:197–222, 1881.
14. Wagner, R.: Die Medianstellung des Stimmbandes bei Recurrenslähmung. Arch. Path. Anat. 120:437–459, 1890.
15. Weeks, C., and Hinton, J. W.: Extralaryngeal division of recurrent laryngeal nerve; its significance in vocal cord paralysis. Ann. Surg. 116:251–258 (Aug.) 1942.

Chapter Four

SURGICAL PATHOLOGY

WILLIAM A. MEISSNER, M.D.

There are numerous occasions when the thyroid surgeon requires a considerable knowledge of thyroid pathology in order to evaluate and to institute proper therapy. Unfortunately the pathology of the thyroid gland is complicated by the great diversity of possible lesions. While some of the pathologic processes are similar to those in other organs, many are different from those seen elsewhere, even in other endocrine glands, and require special study and recognition. In addition, there is a plethora of diagnostic terms, eponyms, and classifications which have added to the problems of understanding the basic pathology. The discussion of pathology in this chapter will emphasize primarily those pathologic changes that are of particular concern in thyroid surgery.

NORMAL GLAND

The normal thyroid gland is bilobed, with the right lobe often being somewhat larger than the left. The two lobes usually are connected by an isthmus, and a midline pyramidal lobe extends upward in about 40 percent of the cases. The isthmus is variable in size and is not always present; one or both of the lateral lobes may be absent from the normal location. In the newborn, the normal thyroid gland averages 1.5 gm.[18] It increases gradually in size until about the age of 16 years, when it reaches its adult weight of 17 gm., plus or minus 7 gm.[32]

The histological work unit of the gland is the follicle[19] (Fig. 4–1). Normal follicles average about 200 μ in diameter. The follicles are lined by a single layer of cuboidal epithelium. The nuclei of the follicular cells are spherical and about one third the diameter of the cell. In various pathologic states, some follicular cells may become larger and develop granular acidophilic cytoplasm and often bizarre, hyperchromatic nuclei. Such cells are called oxyphilic cells (Hürthle cells);[37] their exact significance is unknown. The colloid in the center of the follicle is a glycoprotein (thyroglobulin). The highly vascular stroma surrounding each

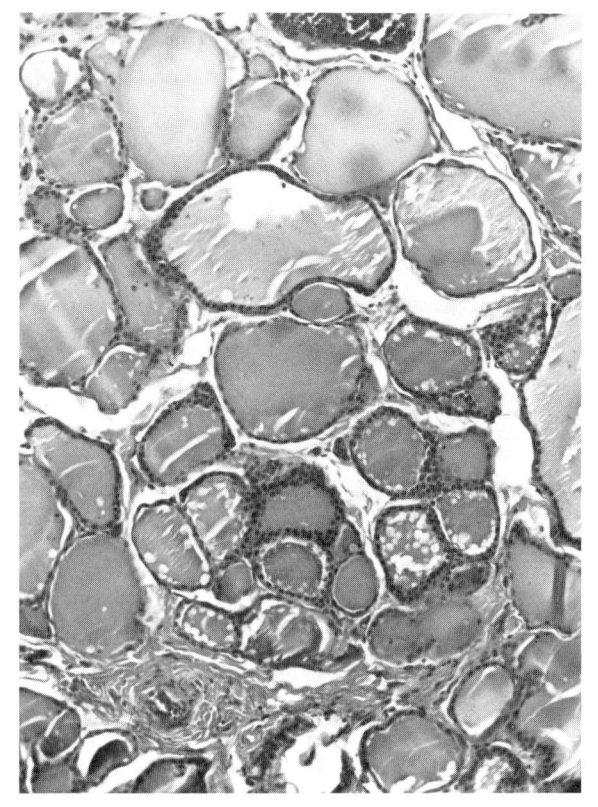

Figure 4-1. Normal thyroid. Low power photomicrograph of thyroid from young adult. (Hematoxylin and eosin, × 130.)

follicle is not prominent except when the gland is congested, as in Graves' disease or heart failure.

The thyroid develops from a tubular downgrowth (thyroglossal duct) from the base of the tongue (foramen caecum). The distal portion of the duct gives rise to the thyroid gland. Normally the remainder of the duct obliterates by the sixth week of embryonic life, but remnants may remain anywhere in the tract—from the base of the tongue to the thyroid gland—giving rise to ectopic nodules of thyroid tissue, cysts, or tumors.[20, 21] Since many tissues descend past the thyroid in embryonic development, fragments of thyroid tissue may be pulled downward with them into an ectopic location such as the mediastinum or pericardium; such ectopic fragments rarely give rise to tumors or cysts.

Occasionally the thyroid anlage partially or completely fails to descend from the base of the tongue, and a lingual thyroid gland develops (Fig. 4-2.). The gland in this location, about the foramen caecum, may develop all the pathologic changes that can be seen in the normally

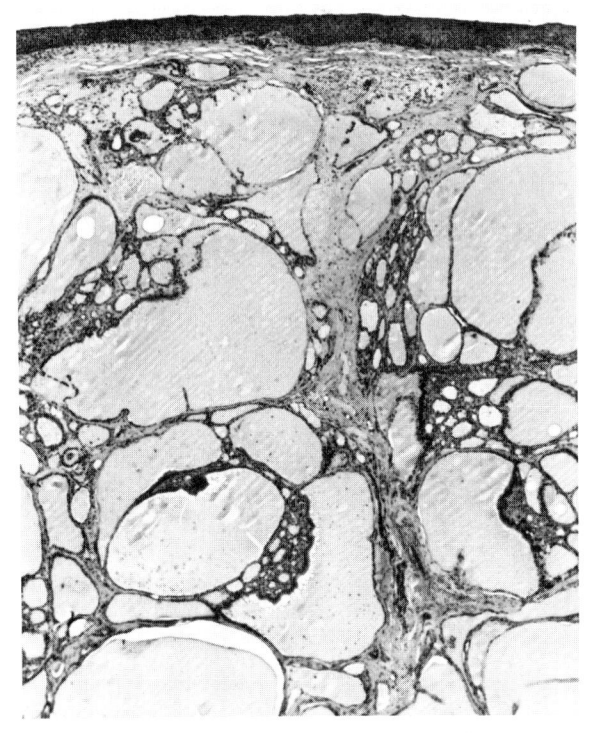

Figure 4–2. Lingual thyroid. The thyroid tissue is covered with squamous epithelium of the tongue and shows typical changes of adenomatous goiter. (Hematoxylin and eosin, × 40.)

located organ, including hyperplasia, adenomatous goiter, and the same spectrum of tumors.

Remnants of the thyroglossal duct may lose or have obstructed their ductal connection with the base of the tongue and become cystic (Fig. 4–3).[36] The cysts, always midline, often have mature thyroid follicles adjacent in the cyst wall. The lining epithelium is columnar, squamous, or embryonic ciliated. The usual range of pathologic processes as seen in the normally located gland is also seen in thyroglossal duct remnants, whether or not associated with a cyst. Tumors of the thyroglossal duct tract are almost exclusively papillary carcinomas.

In many animals the ultimobranchial bodies from the fourth branchial pouch take part in the development of the mature thyroid. It is still debatable whether or not this happens in the human thyroid. The cells of the medullary thyroid carcinoma are thought by some to be of ultimobranchial body origin.

Hyperactivity of the gland and hyperplasia of the follicular epithelium are responses to stimulation by thyroid-stimulating hormone (TSH) of the pituitary. Ordinarily TSH and thyroxin (T4) are in bal-

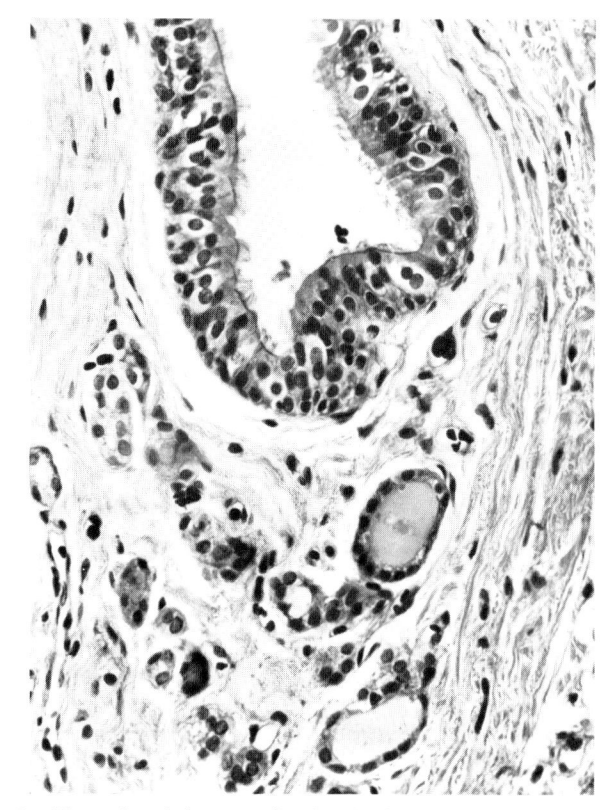

Figure 4–3. Thyroglossal duct cyst lined with ciliated columnar epithelium. Ectopic thyroid follicles lie in adjacent tissues. (Hematoxylin and eosin, × 320.)

ance, so that when T4 diminishes, TSH increases and stimulates the gland to adequate activity to maintain the euthyroid state. With stimulation, the follicles become smaller and contain less colloid, and the epithelium becomes increasingly columnar. As need for hyperactivity decreases, the epithelium diminishes in height, and the follicles return to normal size. With hyperplasia from any cause, there is increased vascularity.

ADENOMATOUS GOITER

The possible causes of inadequate production and secretion of T4 are many. While the commonest cause is a deficiency of iodine in the diet, others include inborn errors of metabolism or any of numerous goitrogenic foods, chemicals, and drugs. No matter what the reason for the deficient output of T4, the gland is stimulated to increased activity (hyperplasia) to maintain the euthyroid state.[2, 47, 48] The resulting hyper-

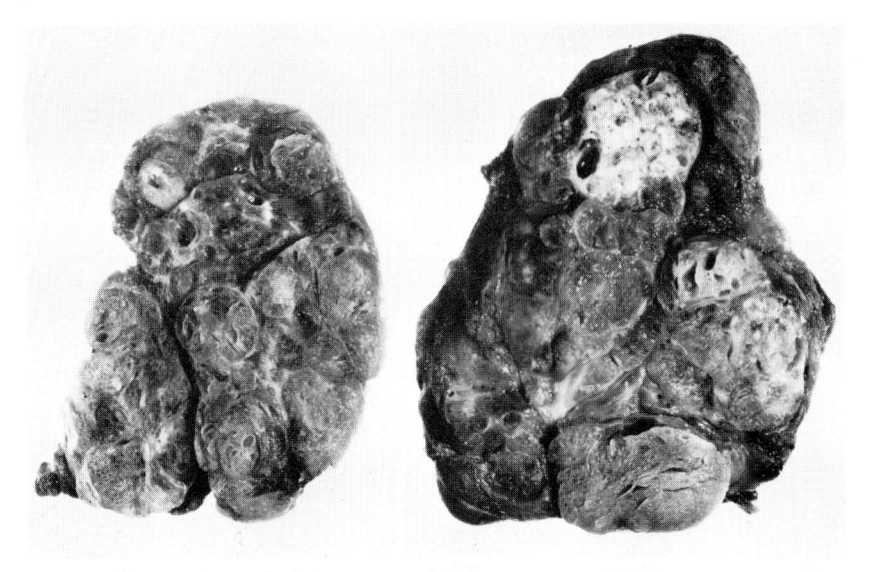

Figure 4-4. Adenomatous goiter removed from a 51-year-old woman. The two lobes together weighed 270 gm. Cut surfaces show multiple nodules of varying size. Some nodules are cystic and some resemble adenomas.

plasia may be mild or intense, depending on the degree of T4 deficiency and resultant TSH stimulation. If the cause of the inadequate secretion of T4 is removed, the gland returns more or less to its normal state. When the cause is intermittent or persists, portions of the gland undergo an "exhaustion atrophy," with the follicles enlarged beyond size and distended with colloid. As the process continues over months and years, the gland becomes progressively enlarged (goitrous), not from the hyperplasia, but because of the enlarged follicles distended with colloid (colloid goiter). With further continuation of the process, some of the large follicles rupture and initiate inflammatory changes. Ultimately various degenerative processes develop, such as hemorrhage, infarction, fibrosis, cyst formation, and calcification. These changes produce multiple nodules (nodular goiter, adenomatous goiter), often resembling tumor (Fig. 4-4).

The macroscopic and microscopic appearance of the thyroid gland in adenomatous goiter varies both with the degree and the duration of the hyperplasia. With intense stimulation by TSH, such as might result, for example, from a severe inborn error of metabolism in the thyroid and a resultant T4 deficiency, the gland becomes diffusely enlarged from an intense hyperplasia, with very tall columnar epithelium and small follicles with little or no colloid. Some goiters in infants are of this type.[22] With low-grade or intermittent stimulation over a long period, as more commonly occurs with iodine deficiency in an endemic goiter area, the significant changes are not those of hyperplasia but rather are of the

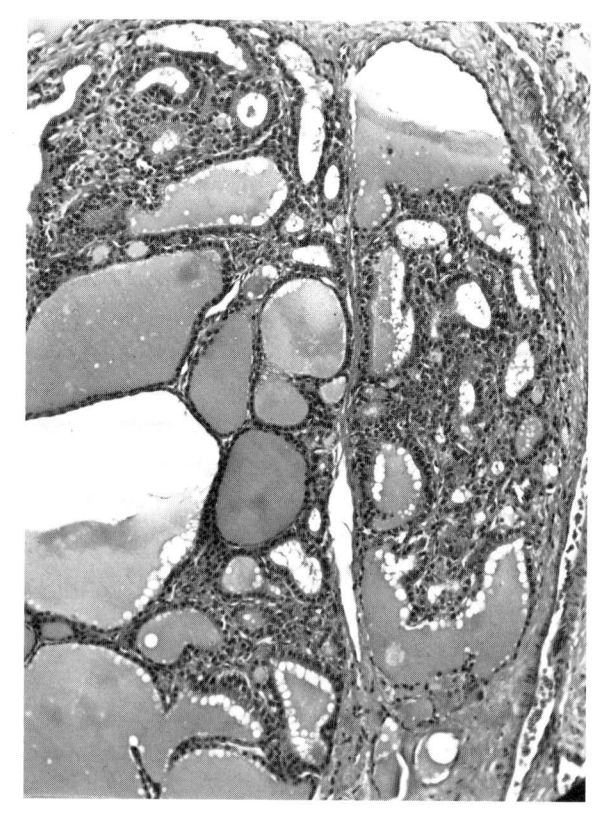

Figure 4-5. Adenomatous goiter. Follicles are often irregular and distended with colloid. Epithelium is focally hyperplastic. (Hematoxylin and eosin, × 130.)

involutional, hyperinvolutional, and degenerative changes secondary to hyperplasia (Figs. 4-5 and 4-6). T4 deficiency from any cause thus produces a goiter which initially is hyperplastic, but which later is characterized by excessive colloid accumulation and which ultimately is multinodular. In the later stages the gland may weigh 1,500 gm. or more, and the degenerative changes are pronounced.

The terms nodular goiter and adenomatous goiter, although often used to encompass the entire process of development, actually refer to the late stages, which are of particular interest to the surgeon. Other terms, such as diffuse colloid goiter, refer to other stages of development; still other terms refer to the underlying cause, such as iodine-deficient goiter and endemic goiter. Unfortunately there is no term in common use that properly encompasses the entire process.

The nodularity of the gland in the later stages of adenomatous goiter is of considerable concern to the surgeon since many of the nodules both clinically and grossly (and at times histologically) resemble a true neoplasm.[50] Tumor nodules, however, are usually solitary and

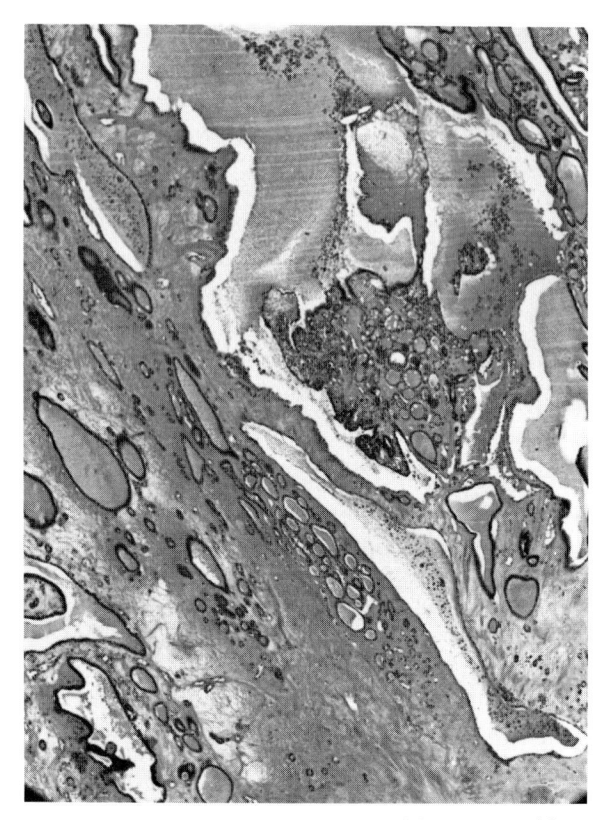

Figure 4–6. Adenomatous goiter. A later stage of the process with great irregularity of follicle shape and size, fibrosis, and hemorrhage. (Hematoxylin and eosin, × 40.)

histologically show more homogeneity of their structure with better encapsulation and more compression of the adjacent gland than do nodules of adenomatous goiter. The distinction can best be made by histological examination.

In addition to compression of adjacent structures by size alone, several other complications may occur, especially in the later stages of adenomatous goiter; for example, one of the nodules may become hyperplastic and secrete excessive hormone, not enough to produce clinical hyperthyroidism but enough to suppress the functional activity of the remainder of the gland. Such "hot" nodules may be autonomous in respect to the homeostatic balance. After a time the nodule may involute from its hyperactivity and another nodule or nodules may become "hot" for a variable period of time.

Another complication arises when much of the gland, not just one nodule, becomes hyperactive and autonomous to produce clinical hyperthyroidism, often called secondary hyperthyroidism to distinguish it from the primary hyperthyroidism of Graves' disease.[31] Such a gland produces relatively mild hyperthyroidism and never has exophthalmos associated with it.

Although theoretical and experimental data suggest that the factors causing development of adenomatous goiter (excessive TSH stimulation) are the same as those that produce thyroid carcinoma, in actual practice and in careful statistical studies of incidence, adenomatous goiter is, at most, only a mildly precancerous condition.

PRIMARY HYPERPLASIA

Synonyms for primary hyperplasia include Graves' disease, Basedow's disease, primary hyperthyroidism, diffuse toxic goiter, and exophthalmic goiter.

Primary hyperplasia is a systemic disorder manifesting principally as a severe thyroid hyperplasia with clinical hyperthyroidism and often an accompanying exophthalmos. Some patients, in addition, have hyperplasia of the thymus and other lymphoid tissues. The hyperplasia of the thyroid is not produced by TSH stimulation, as in adenomatous goiter, but by another factor or factors (possibly long-acting thyroid stimulator) which are independent of the usual homeostatic mechanisms.

Macroscopically the thyroid gland is diffusely enlarged, meaty, and intensely hyperemic. The weight usually is three to four times normal. The capsule is smooth, and there is no nodularity.

Histologically the hyperplastic follicular epithelium is tall columnar and often extends as papillary infoldings into the follicular lumen. The follicles are small and have little colloid. All portions of the gland are involved to a similar degree (Fig. 4–7).

With involution the gland becomes smaller and the hyperemia diminishes, making surgery more feasible, and the follicular epithelium and follicles as well as the colloid content return more or less to the normal state. However, with repeated bouts or with longstanding disease, some follicles may undergo hyperinvolution with excessive colloid accumulation and thus enter a phase of development of adenomatous goiter. Involution may occur spontaneously or may be induced by iodine or irradiation; in any event, the involutionary changes are similar. Preparations of thiouracil used to bring about euthyroidism before operation do not produce specific changes, although glands from patients so treated often appear histologically more hyperplastic than their clinical thyroid state would indicate.

In Graves' disease many thyroid glands show an infiltration of lymphocytes, varying from a scattering of lymphocytes to the formation of actual secondary germinal centers. The infiltrate does not correlate with age, sex, degree or duration of hyperthyroidism, or with preoperative therapy. The infiltrate often remains after the hyperplasia has

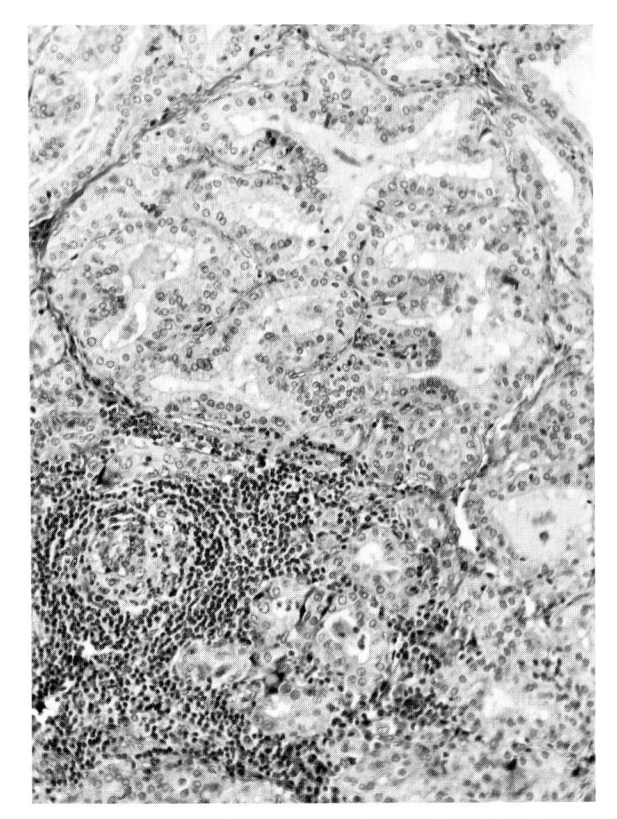

Figure 4-7. Graves' disease. The patient, a 16-year-old girl, had hyperthyroidism and exophthalmos for five months. Small follicles are lined with tall columnar epithelium, often arranged in papillary fronds. The focus of lymphocyte infiltration is a common accompaniment of hyperplasia. (Hematoxylin and eosin, × 150.)

involuted, giving the appearance of a nonspecific chronic thyroiditis. Hyperplasia of the thymus, lymph nodes, and spleen and lymphocytosis may all be found in Graves' disease.

Another frequently associated condition is ophthalmopathy, which is produced by edema, hypertrophy, cellular infiltration, and fibrosis of the retro-orbital muscles and fat. It occasionally is seen in patients who are euthyroid by all the usual laboratory tests of thyroid function. The exophthalmos may persist or even may progress after alleviation of the hyperthyroidism by any current method of treatment, although in the majority of cases it improves.

Pretibial edema occurs in some patients with Graves' disease, usually in association with ophthalmopathy. It consists of a mucopolysaccharide deposit in the subcutaneous tissues. Most commonly it occurs in the lower legs and feet, but may also involve hands, forearms, and even the cheeks and orbits.

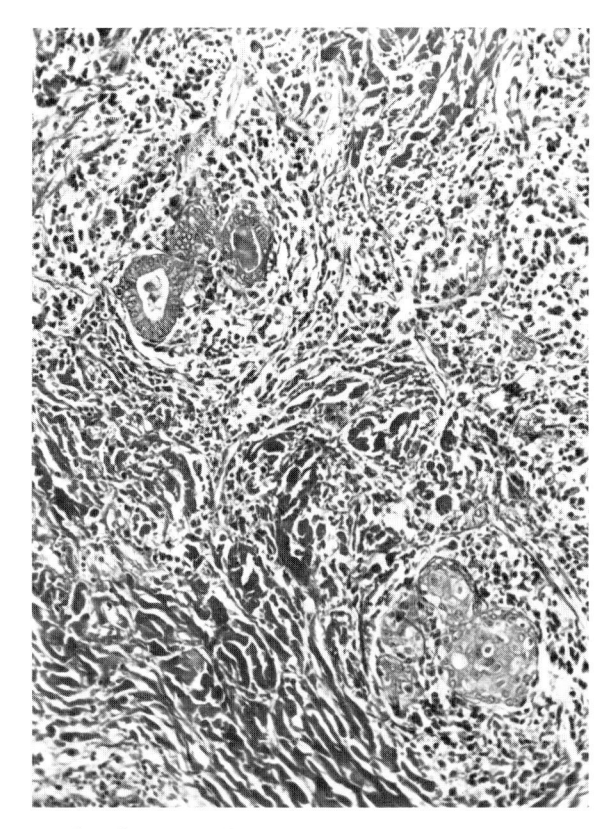

Figure 4-8. Chronic nonspecific thyroiditis in a 53-year-old man. In this advanced stage there is much fibrosis In addition to the inflammatory cell infiltrate. The residual follicles are distorted and some epithelium shows squamous metaplasia. (Hematoxylin and eosin, × 130.)

THYROIDITIS

Acute pyogenic thyroiditis is infrequent. Furthermore, thyroiditis in specific diseases, such as tuberculosis or syphilis, is also quite rare.

Chronic Nonspecific Thyroiditis

The commonest type of inflammation of the thyroid is chronic and nonspecific. In this type the amount of fibrosis is variable, with an infiltrate of inflammatory cells, chiefly lymphocytes and plasma cells (Fig. 4-8). The gland may be focally or rather diffusely involved, and the gland sometimes is enlarged up to 100 gm. or more. The process may be mistaken for tumor because of firmness, nodularity, or adherence to adjacent structures. Although the etiology of any single case is usually unclear, chronic nonspecific thyroiditis probably represents the effect of any of a number of causes, such as trauma, vascular insufficiency, previous hyperplasia, and irradiation or auto-immunity, or both.

Three types of thyroiditis that are more or less distinctive and usually can be differentiated from the chronic nonspecific type are subacute thyroiditis, invasive fibrous thyroiditis (Riedel's struma), and struma lymphomatosa (Hashimoto's disease).

Subacute Thyroiditis

Subacute thyroiditis, also called viral, granulomatous, pseudotuberculous, or de Quervain's thyroiditis, is probably of viral origin.[12] Clinical symptoms of tenderness of the gland of a few weeks' or months' duration (subacute) bring the patient in for medical advice, and a localized firmness of the gland is palpated. Usually only a portion of one lobe is involved, although the process may be more generalized and progressive. The involved focus is firm, poorly demarcated, and yellow-brown. Histologically the disease is characteristic and easily recognized, either in tissue from a needle biopsy or from a formal biopsy resection, and the diagnosis may be made by frozen section. Many follicles contain inflammatory cells which, in the earlier stages, are principally polymorphonuclears. Later, colloid is broken down in the involved follicles and ingested by foreign body giant cells which, by being centered in the follicles, give the appearance of a tubercle. The tissue between the follicles also shows variable amounts of round cell inflammatory infiltrate and fibrosis (Fig. 4–9).

Subacute thyroiditis is a self-limited process and responds well to medical management, so the only indication for surgery is biopsy (needle biopsy is adequate) to confirm the clinical impression. With healing, the gland shows surprisingly little in the way of residual damage, although some cases of nonspecific chronic thyroiditis may represent the residuum of subacute thyroiditis.

Invasive Fibrous Thyroiditis (Riedel's Struma)

Invasive fibrous thyroiditis is a rare condition in which there is an inflammatory infiltrate with dense fibrous tissue involving a portion of the thyroid gland and extending through its capsule into the adjacent structures.[55] Similar invasive fibrous tissue deposits are seen in the mediastinum and elsewhere, sometimes in the same patient with the thyroid involvement, and it seems likely that the condition is not primarily or solely one of the thyroid. At any rate, when the thyroid is involved, the firmness and fixation are, of course, suggestive of cancer, and a biopsy or resection is usually done. Simple focal fibrosis, occurring secondarily in adenomatous goiter or in chronic nonspecific thyroiditis, is not invasive and should not be diagnosed as Riedel's struma.

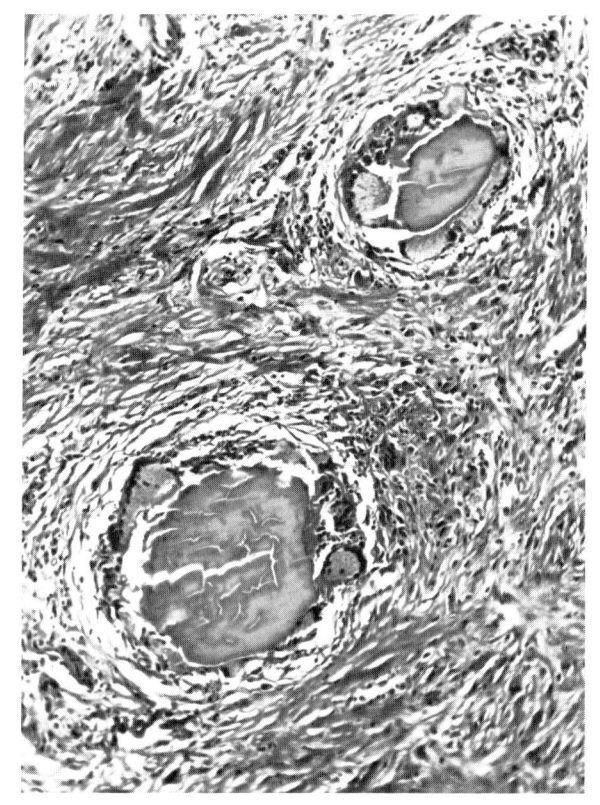

Figure 4-9 Subacute thyroiditis. Two clusters of colloid representing broken-down follicles are surrounded by foreign body giant cells. Stroma is fibrotic. (Hematoxylin and eosin, × 130.)

Struma Lymphomatosa

Synonyms for struma lymphomatosa are Hashimoto's disease, autoimmune thyroiditis, and lymphocytic thyroiditis (some types).[53] Struma lymphomatosa is characterized by a diffuse enlargement of the gland to as much as several hundred grams, but a weight of 50 to 100 gm. is more common. The gland is lobulated, and the capsule is not adherent. The cut surface is yellow-brown, resembling a lymph node involved with lymphosarcoma.

Histologically the follicles are smaller than normal size, and much of the follicular epithelium is acidophilic (Fig. 4-10). Colloid is scanty. Between the follicles is an infiltrate of lymphocytes and plasma cells; secondary lymphoid nodules frequently are formed. In some types of Hashimoto's disease there may be, in addition, considerable stromal fibrosis. From a biopsy or examination of one portion of the gland alone it is not possible to make a pathologic diagnosis of struma lymphomatosa, since changes of nonspecific chronic thyroiditis may be focally

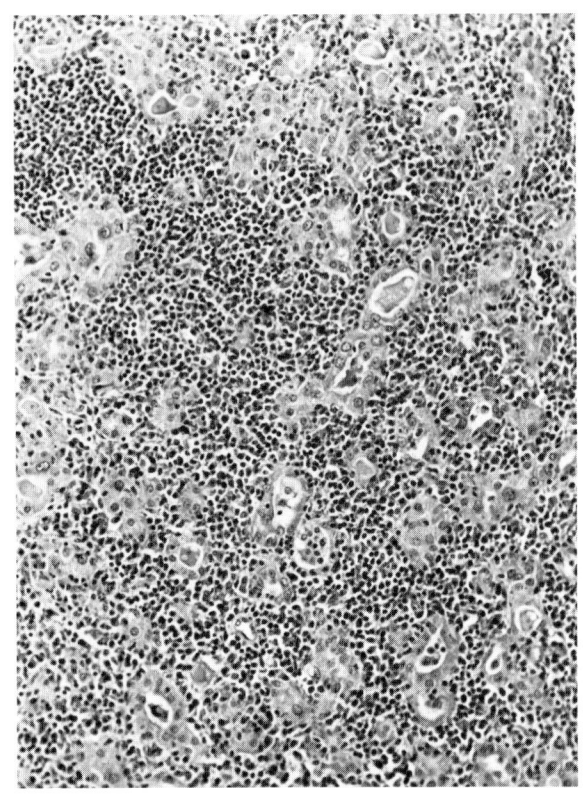

Figure 4-10. Hashimoto's disease. The follicles are small and contain little colloid. The cellular infiltrate in the stroma consists of lymphocytes and plasma cells. (Hematoxylin and eosin, × 130.)

very similar. The diffuseness of the involvement of the entire gland is very important in the diagnosis.

Since antithyroid antibodies are almost always demonstrable in patients with struma lymphomatosa and are found more frequently than in any other thyroid disease, the condition is thought to represent an autoimmune process. It occurs predominantly in women, especially between the ages of 40 and 60 years.

Complications include pressure from size and adjacent neck structures. Hypothyroidism is common. While a few instances of carcinoma and lymphoma have been reported arising in glands with struma lymphomatosa, at the most it should be considered only a minimal precancerous condition. More important is its confusion with tumor clinically, especially in the type with considerable fibrosis.

BENIGN TUMORS

Except for the rare teratoma of the thyroid,[41] which usually presents in the newborn or during early infancy, benign tumors of the thyroid

Surgical Pathology 37

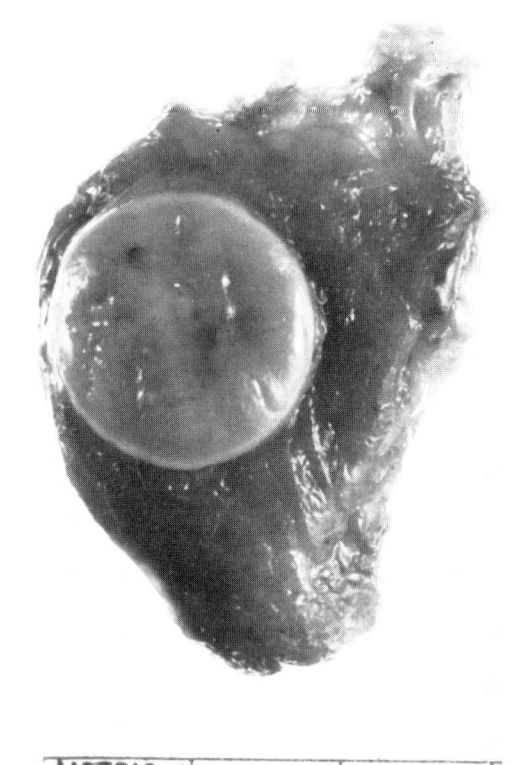

Figure 4-11. Follicular adenoma. The solitary nodule in an otherwise normal gland is distinctly encapsulated. In the center of the tumor are early degenerative changes.

are, for practical purposes, of epithelial origin and, thus, adenomas.[28] Although an occasional adenoma shows papillary structure, nearly all are follicular. The problems of benign tumors of the thyroid are concerned with follicular adenomas.

Follicular adenomas may be, and often are, subclassified into many different categories, depending upon whether the follicles are small (embryonal, fetal, microfollicular), large (colloid, macrofollicular), whether the cells are oxyphilic (oxyphil, Hürthle cell) or the structure is not typical of any of the above (atypical).[13] Such detailed subclassifications are of little practical value, and the term follicular adenoma is sufficient and simple with the exception of the atypical variant and, to a lesser degree, the small follicle variant, since these are more difficult to differentiate from invasive tumor (carcinoma) without multiple sections for histological study.

Macroscopically the follicular adenoma is an encapsulated, round-to-ovoid mass of variable size (Fig. 4-11.). The consistency and cut surface vary greatly with the extent of degenerative changes. Such changes (hemorrhage, infarction, cyst formation, fibrosis, and calcification) are

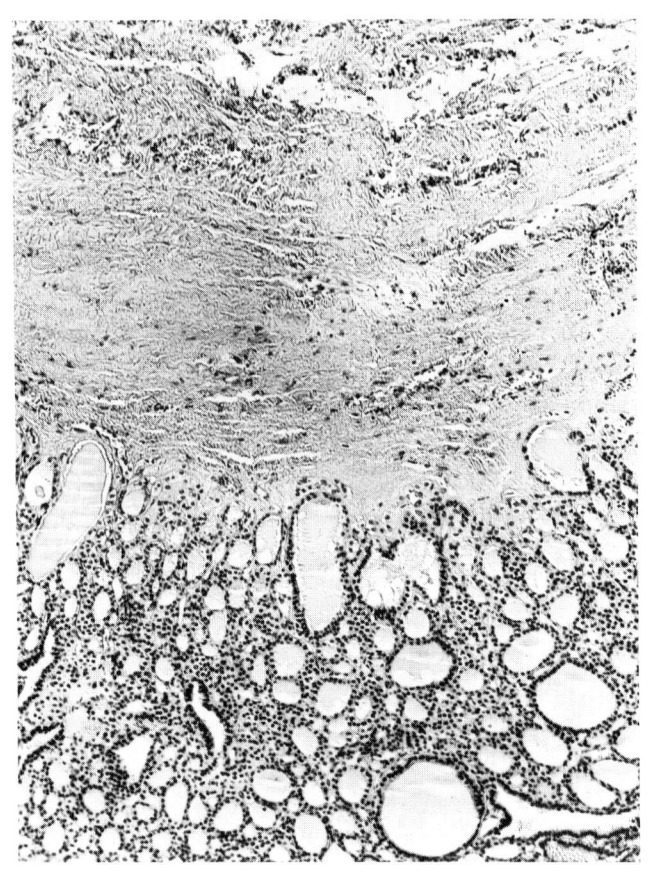

Figure 4–12. Follicular adenoma. The follicle-forming tumor is well demarcated from the compressed adjacent gland by a fibrous capsule. (Hematoxylin and eosin, × 100.)

frequent and are similar to those seen in adenomatous goiter. Often acute hemorrhage or infarction causes an alarming sudden enlargement for which the patient seeks medical advice. The distinction between adenoma and a nodule of adenomatous goiter by clinical or macroscopic examination may be difficult or impossible. In an otherwise normal-appearing gland, a solitary circumscribed nodule is usually an adenoma rather than an adenomatous goiter.

The microscopic appearance of follicular adenoma varies with the cell type and the follicular size as described. In addition, the degenerative changes seen are even more conspicuous. The true adenoma in addition to being *solitary* shows a *relatively uniform structure* that is *different from the remainder* of the gland, a *complete capsule*, and *compression of the adjacent gland* (Fig. 4–12). Although one or more of these criteria may be present in an adenomatous nodule, they are usually not so prominent or well developed as in the true follicular adenoma. Particular care must be taken to exclude an early stage of carcinoma in a lesion appearing to be adenoma by searching for microscopic evidence of malignant tumor, such as capsular or blood vessel invasion. This search is especially important in atypical and microfollicular adenomas.

In addition to the frequent degenerative changes, there are other possible complications. If the adenoma is large, it may compress structures adjacent to the thyroid. Another infrequent complication is hyperthyroidism. While follicular adenomas often function to a degree and will take up some radioiodine, they rarely hyperfunction to a degree sufficient to produce hyperthyroidism.[6] The "hot" nodule, with few exceptions, is a nodule of adenomatous goiter rather than a true neoplasm. Transition from benign adenoma to cancer is another possible complication but, except in the case of some giant cell carcinomas, is difficult to prove. It seems likely from available evidence that most adenomas remain benign and that most carcinomas are malignant from their inception. The difficulty in adequately assessing the concept arises partly from the fact that the only macroscopic or microscopic difference between an adenoma and some carcinomas is the presence of minimal invasion of capsule, or invasion of blood vessels or lymphatic vessels.

MALIGNANT TUMORS

Meaningful data on the occurrence of thyroid cancer are difficult to obtain. Evaluations based on study of surgical specimens are of questionable value because of patient selection. Incidence studies based on autopsy material include a high number of occult carcinomas, many of which perhaps remain dormant indefinitely unless "promoted" by factors still poorly understood. The autopsy incidence in a meticulous study by Silverberg and Vidone[44] was 1.79 percent in unselected cases. Haber et al.[11] found the incidence in Hawaii to be much higher than on the mainland and particularly high in Chinese women. Recent autopsy studies on Japanese have shown, when very minute papillary cancers are included, an incidence of about 20 percent.[38] The number of cases of cancer of the thyroid in the United States seems to be increasing and, according to one report, has doubled in the last two decades.[3] Death from thyroid carcinoma is uncommon—about 1,100 per year in the United States.[9]

Both benign and malignant tumors of the thyroid can readily be induced in laboratory animals by factors resulting in excessive TSH secretion (goitrogenic drugs, hemithyroidectomy, irradiation to the thyroid) and by TSH itself.[46] In man, causative factors are unclear, and all types of associated or preexisting thyroid disease have been implicated but none to a very noteworthy degree. Exposure of the thyroid to ionizing radiation in infancy and early childhood is one factor of definite significance[5] and is well documented in studies of Winship and Rosvoll,[52] who

Table 4-1. Classification of Thyroid Tumors

>   Benign
>   Adenoma
>   Teratoma
>   Malignant
>   Papillary adenocarcinoma
>   Follicular carcinoma
>   Medullary carcinoma
>   Undifferentiated carcinoma
>   Lymphoma
>   Secondary tumor

found that in the majority of cases of childhood thyroid cancer there had been radiation exposure. Whether or not related to previous exposure to radiation, cancer of the thyroid in children and young adults runs a slow clinical course even in the presence of clinical metastases.

The histological classification of thyroid cancer (Table 4-1) effectively grades the degree of malignancy of the respective tumors. The papillary adenocarcinoma is extremely low grade, the follicular more highly malignant, the medullary even more so, and the undifferentiated thyroid carcinomas are among the most malignant of any cancers of any tissue. While prognosis relates very well with the histological type, the presence of remote metastases and of direct extension of the tumor into adjacent neck structures are also important in assessing prognosis on an individual patient.[16, 43] Metastases in cervical lymph nodes are of less prognostic significance.

Small accumulations of normal-appearing thyroid follicles are occasional incidental findings in cervical lymph nodes.[30] The nests are neither visible nor palpable. The epithelium is not papillary. While the finding of such nests always raises the question of cancer, current opinion is that they represent non-neoplastic extensions by the process of "benign metastasis" of normal thyroid tissue from the main gland. If, however, the nests are large enough to be visible or palpable or if the epithelium is papillary, then tumor metastasis from a primary carcinoma in the main gland must be anticipated.

Frozen section at the time of operation may be of considerable value to the surgeon. It must be remembered, however, that some minimal carcinomas may show invasive characteristics at only a few foci in their capsule and that such invasion may not be identified without study of numerous sections, rarely possible at time of frozen section. Most benign processes can be distinguished easily from cancer with frozen sections, and the general type of tumor can usually be recognized. Frozen section may also be of considerable value in assisting in the evaluation of the presence of tumor in lymph nodes. Needle biopsy is primarily of value in confirming the diagnosis of cancer in what appears clinically to be an inoperable lesion. It has not been a feasible technique in the diagnosis of

SURGICAL PATHOLOGY 41

Figure 4–13. Papillary carcinoma. The cut surface of the right lobe shows a lobulated, pale tumor which replaces about one half of the lobe. The patient was a 37-year-old woman who had been treated with desiccated thyroid for one year in an attempt to suppress a palpable nodule which continued to enlarge.

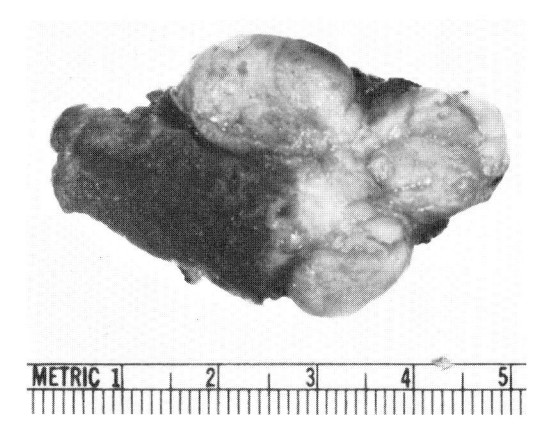

differentiated cancers because of the possibility of implantation. Neither has it been useful in the diagnosis of benign tumors or Hashimoto's disease.

Papillary Carcinoma

Papillary carcinoma is the commonest type of thyroid cancer.[24] It occurs in all age groups and characteristically runs a slow clinical course which corresponds well to its histological evidence of activity.

Papillary carcinomas present as irregular, solid, or cystic (cystadenocarcinoma) masses (Fig. 4–13). The cut surface is rough, and calcium deposits are frequently present, sometimes so extensive as to mask the true nature of the lesion. The content of the cysts, if such are present, is brown, watery fluid.

Histologically the tumor is composed of papillary fronds of epithelium (Fig. 4–14). The cells are usually in a single layer lining the connective tissue stalks, which are quite vascular. The individual columnar cells are relatively uniform, have amphophilic cytoplasm, and resemble mildly hyperplastic thyroid epithelium, but with a less orderly arrangement. The nuclei also are quite uniform and often have a ground-glass appearance; they are seldom hyperchromatic and only rarely have demonstrable mitoses.

In some papillary carcinomas there are rounded calcific deposits (psammoma bodies) scattered throughout but particularly prominent in stroma of the stalks of fronds (Fig. 4–15). The presence of psammoma bodies is highly characteristic of papillary carcinoma, but they are seen occasionally in other thyroid tumors and even in non-neoplastic conditions; furthermore, not all papillary tumors contain psammoma bodies. Their significance is unknown. The bodies sometimes are found without accompanying tumor cells as deposits in the gland or in lymph nodes.

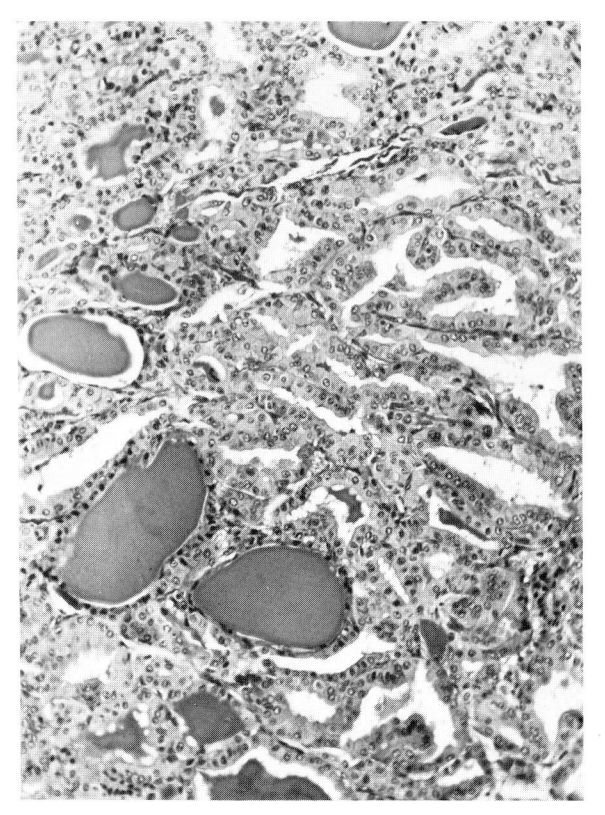

Figure 4–14. Papillary carcinoma. The tumor was removed from a 65-year-old woman who had had hoarseness for one year. It predominantly forms papillary processes, but there is also an admixture of colloid-filled follicles (mixed papillary and follicular carcinoma). (Hematoxylin and eosin, × 130.)

Such "naked" psammoma bodies probably represent extension or metastasis of papillary carcinoma at some time in the past, with the tumor cells dying off and leaving the calcific remains behind.

There are, of course, numerous variants to the histologic pattern of classic papillary carcinoma. Calcification, other than psammoma bodies, is common, as is cyst formation by the tumor. Some papillary carcinomas, especially in younger patients, have a rather solid pattern, with the papilliferous structures less well developed. Still others have a mixture of follicular elements and, indeed, pure papillary carcinoma without follicular components is uncommon.

As with most thyroid cancers, papillary carcinoma is more common in women at a ratio of about 3 to 1. Papillary carcinoma may be found at any age. The incidence does not increase much with increasing age, as is the case in other thyroid cancers. The tumor often shows invasion, both of lymphatic and blood vessels; however, metastases resulting from blood vessel dissemination are infrequent, with the tumor rarely metas-

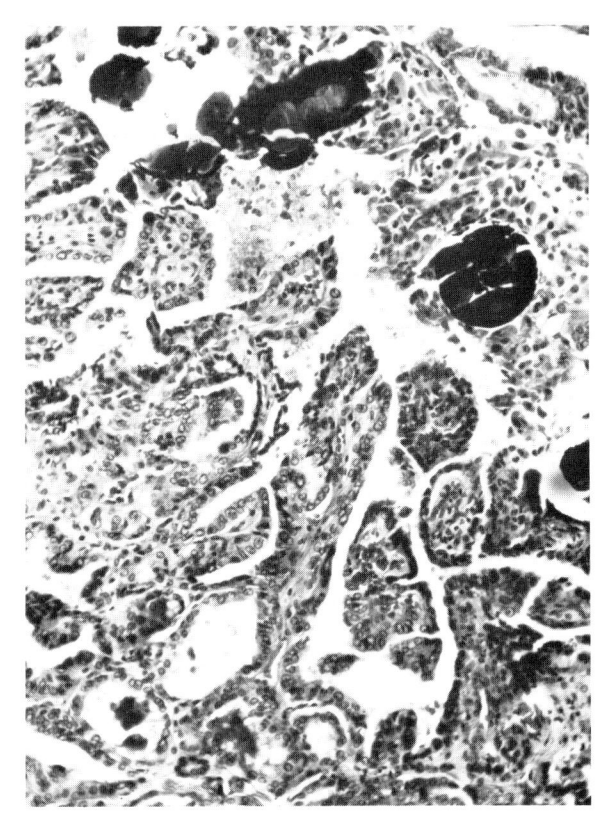

Figure 1-15. Papillary carcinoma removed from a 26-year-old woman. A firm nodule, 1.5 cm., was discovered by palpation during routine physical examination. In this tumor the follicular components are less conspicuous and there are typical psammoma bodies. (Hematoxylin and eosin, × 130.)

tasizing to lung, bone, brain, or other viscera. Lymphatic metastases to the cervical lymph nodes are very common, however, and the tumor in the nodes shows the same histologic pattern and slow clinical growth as in the primary lesion. In some patients the lymph nodes seem to offer better soil for tumor growth, resulting in the lymph node metastasis becoming much larger than the primary tumor and, indeed, even presenting as the initial finding of tumor. A papillary carcinoma in a cervical lymph node represents metastatic disease from a primary tumor in the main gland, even if one cannot be palpated there. Papillary carcinomas do not arise in lymph nodes; "carcinomas arising in lateral aberrant thyroid" are metastases. Even distant metastases occasionally occur from very small occult carcinomas. Patchefsky et al.[33] reported a large metastatic growth to a vertebra from an occult sclerosing cancer 0.85 cm. in diameter. Sampson et al.[39] define an occult cancer as being a tumor, usually papillary, not clinically suspected, and 1.5 cm. or less in diameter. Occult cancers are often partially sclerosed.

More important than involvement of cervical lymph nodes in respect to prognosis is the local growth of the tumor. When the tumor extends beyond the thyroid capsule, the prognosis becomes considerably poorer.[54] Although not common, such direct extensions may invade any of the adjacent tissues, including the esophagus, trachea, and recurrent laryngeal nerves.

Another potential of the papillary carcinoma is transition to a more malignant, often highly malignant, neoplasm such as a giant cell carcinoma.[15] Most papillary carcinomas that persist remain relatively consistent in their structural pattern throughout a long course.[25] Their transition to a more malignant tumor, however, remains a constant threat so long as residual tumor is present. Death from papillary thyroid carcinoma usually is the result of the tumor increasing its malignant potential—a development that may not occur until after 20 or 30 years of tumor persistence.

The tumor grows so slowly that five-year survival rates are almost meaningless. The 10-year survival rate is about 80 percent.[54] (Fatal termination, however, can occur within three to five years after diagnosis.) In fatal cases,[49] death was caused about equally by local recurrence or by distant metastasis to lungs, brain, or bone.

FOLLICULAR CARCINOMA

Follicular carcinoma belongs in the group of differentiated cancers of the thyroid and runs a low-grade clinical course. It is the second most common cancer type.

Follicular carcinomas may appear encapsulated or may extend by obvious macroscopic invasion into adjacent gland and adjacent structures. When the amount of invasion is localized, the tumor resembles, and may be indistinguishable grossly from, a follicular adenoma or an adenomatous nodule. Similar degenerative changes occur in all three of these lesions, such as hemorrhage, infarction, cyst formation, fibrosis, and calcification. Since the differentiation of thyroid carcinoma from a benign nodule is often difficult from clinical or macroscopic findings, one of the main reasons for removal of a thyroid nodule is to allow histological examination to confirm or to exclude the diagnosis of cancer.

Histologically follicular carcinomas show structural patterns comparable to those seen in benign follicular adenomas—microfollicular, macrofollicular, and so forth.[26] The important histological finding for the diagnosis of carcinoma is invasion—invasion of capsule, adjacent gland, and lymphatic or blood vessels (Fig. 4-16). Since some follicular carcinomas are so well differentiated they resemble normal thyroid tissues, examination of the center of a nodule is not particularly rewarding because invasion is not evident here. It is the periphery of the nod-

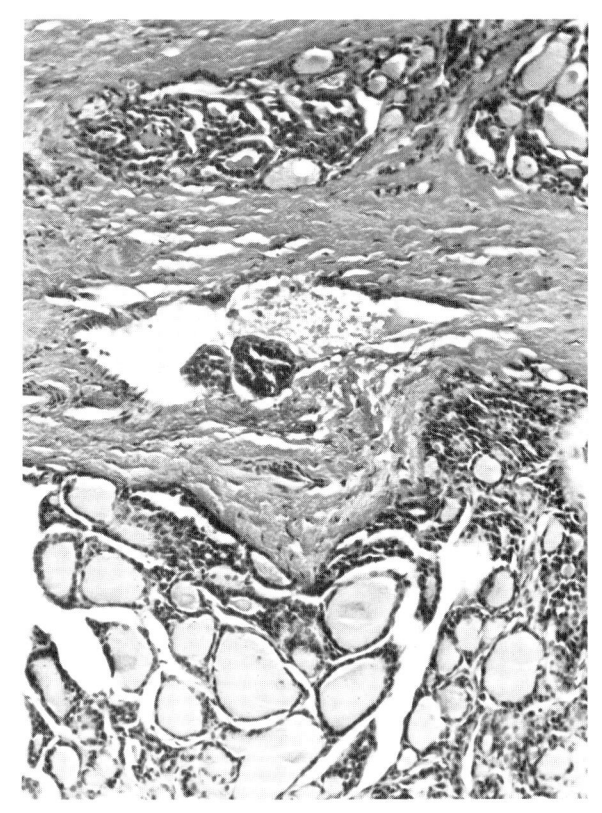

Figure 4-16 Follicular carcinoma. The tumor was a cold nodule in a 22-year-old woman. It is well differentiated, forming numerous follicles. There is extension of the tumor through the capsule into the adjacent gland and tumor has invaded the blood vessel in the center of the photograph. (Hematoxylin and eosin, × 130.)

ule that should be examined carefully, since it is in this location that invasion can best be discovered either by extension into the capsule or by direct invasion of blood vessels or adjacent gland. With better developed cancers, the invasion is seen macroscopically, and such careful histological search is unnecessary.

There are variants and subtypes of follicular carcinomas, most of which, however, are of little importance in prognosis and treatment. For example, some or all of the cells in the tumor may be oxyphilic (Hürthle cells). In other tumors the cells may have a clear cytoplasm resembling renal cell carcinoma. A mixture with papillary elements, as noted before, is common, and only a relatively small proportion of follicular carcinomas are purely follicular. The mixture of these two elements is so common that the term "mixed" papillary and follicular carcinoma has gained considerable usage. It is true that most such mixed carcinomas are very low grade and behave as papillary carcinomas so far as prognosis is concerned. A follicular component should always be mentioned in the diagnosis of a thyroid cancer since it may be important in helping to evaluate subsequent use of radioiodine in therapy. Follicular carcinomas take up radioiodine more avidly than do papillary carcinomas or any other thyroid cancer.

Follicular carcinoma occurs in all age groups. It is more common in women than in men. These tumors at times remain well circumscribed for long periods with only minimal invasion. Other tumors are much more aggressive and invade the adjacent thyroid structures and extend into the adjacent neck in an early stage of their growth. Blood vessel invasion and lymphatic vessel invasion are both frequent, and both blood-borne metastases and lymph node metastases are common. Tumors showing only minimal invasion and appearing grossly as benign tumors may, nevertheless, metastasize to lung, bone, or brain. The distant metastases may not become evident for many years after removal of the primary tumor.

As with papillary carcinoma, a transition to a more malignant form of tumor, such as giant cell cancer, is always a potential as long as residual tumor remains.

Since follicular carcinomas more closely resemble the structure of the normal thyroid than any other thyroid cancer, it is not surprising that they may take up iodine in sufficient amounts to warrant use of radioiodine in the treatment of metastases or even the primary tumor itself.[34] It should be remembered, however, that seldom does a tumor take up iodine as avidly as the normal gland, and ablation of the entire gland is necessary for radioiodine therapy to be effective. Most follicular tumors are "cold" nodules, but nevertheless quite capable of taking up iodine if they are not competing with the normal gland. Hyperthyroidism from excessive activity of a follicular carcinoma is rare.

The prognosis of follicular carcinoma depends largely on the stage (extent of invasion) at the time of therapy. With minimal invasion, the prognosis is very good, but with more extension the five-year survival is less than 50 percent. Overall five-year survival is about 65 percent.[17] In patients dying from follicular carcinoma,[42] 89 percent had lymph node metastasis, 56 percent had lung metastasis, and 17 percent had metastasis to bone, brain, or liver.

MEDULLARY CARCINOMA

Medullary carcinoma is a recently recognized and defined cancer.[14,51] It is midway in degree of malignancy between the differentiated and undifferentiated carcinomas. It has a characteristic stroma that stains for amyloid.[1] It accounts for 5 to 10 percent of primary thyroid cancers.

Medullary carcinoma presents as an ill defined, nonencapsulated, solid, invasive mass. The tumor usually is extremely firm. At the time of presentation clinically, the mass in the thyroid may already be fixed to adjacent structures.

SURGICAL PATHOLOGY 47

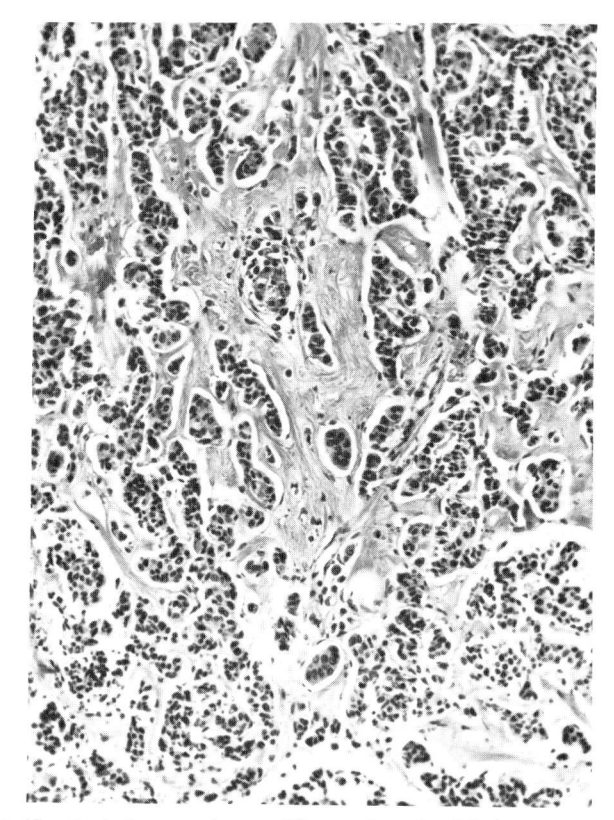

Figure 4-17. Medullary carcinoma. The cords and solid clusters of tumor cells are surrounded by a stroma containing amyloid. The tumor in the 64-year-old woman was inoperable, and only a biopsy specimen was taken. (Hematoxylin and eosin, × 130.)

Histologically the tumor is characteristic, being composed of masses or columns of epithelial cells lying in a dense stroma that stains typically for amyloid (Fig. 4-17). The tumor cells are round or polygonal or even spindle shaped; hyperchromatic nuclei are frequent, and mitoses are often present. The pattern of the tumor cells does not vary much in an individual tumor, but several possible patterns of growth may be found, such as one resembling carcinoid, one resembling chemodectoma, and one having a trabecular pattern. Formation of follicles is occasionally seen, but it is doubtful if true colloid is formed by the tumor. Tumor cells form the amyloid that is deposited in the stroma, and sometimes amyloid may be seen lying within the cytoplasm of the tumor cells. The amyloid, since it is formed by the tumor itself, is found in metastases as well as in the primary neoplasm. Whether amyloid must necessarily be present to allow the diagnosis of medullary carcinoma is still debatable. Polliack and Freund[35] have reported amyloid stroma in a mixed papillary and follicular carcinoma.

Medullary carcinoma is rare in children but occurs in adults of all ages and is more common in older persons. Again, as in other thyroid cancers, it is more frequent in women than in men. It is a familial tumor and may be associated with pheochromocytomas, hyperplasia of the parathyroid glands, carcinoid tumors, and neuromas of the gastrointestinal tract (Sipple's syndrome).[4] There is a close relationship to neurofibromatosis. Calcitonin is produced by the tumor and may be demonstrated in the blood or urine of a patient with the cancer even before the tumor is palpable in the thyroid. Melvin et al.,[29] by radioimmunoassay, determined serum and urine calcitonin levels in 83 members of a family with four known medullary carcinomas. Twelve showing elevated levels of calcitonin underwent thyroidectomy, and each showed bilateral medullary carcinomas ranging from "microscopic" size to 1.4 cm.; six already had metastasis to cervical lymph nodes.

Medullary carcinoma characteristically pursues a low-grade but progressive course, with local invasive growth into adjacent structures and with metastases both to cervical lymph nodes and to distant locations. The metastases contain amyloid and form calcitonin just as the primary tumor.[7]

The prognosis is relatively poor, but not so bad as with the undifferentiated cancers. Freeman and Lindsay[10] reported a series of 33 cases in which 13 patients died from the cancer. In 20 autopsied cases[51] there were 13 instances of metastases in lymph nodes, nine in lungs, five in liver, four in bones, and four in adrenals. Death occurs either from local extension of disease in the neck or from disseminated metastases.

UNDIFFERENTIATED CARCINOMA

The undifferentiated carcinomas are those that show either no or relatively few differentiated structures, such as papillae or follicles, and do not form amyloid stroma. The tumors often resemble sarcoma more than carcinoma in their cellular structure, and the epithelial nature may be difficult to demonstrate even after examining numerous foci of tumor. The tumors as a class grow rapidly, are highly malignant, and are often inoperable at the time of presentation because of extensive invasion of adjacent neck structures. The undifferentiated carcinomas may be subdivided into those composed of small or smaller cells and those composed of spindle or giant cells, the latter being more malignant.

The undifferentiated carcinomas with small or relatively *small cells* may grow either in a compact or a diffuse fashion.[27] The compact small cell tumors often lie in a dense hyaline stroma and suggest the possibility that they may be variants of medullary carcinoma but without amyloid stroma.

The structural pattern of the tumor cells is nondescript, although

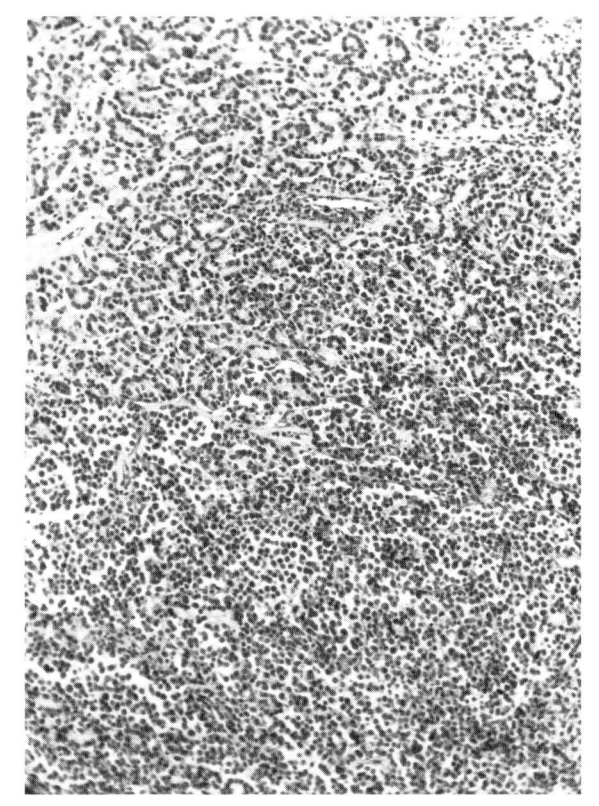

Figure 4-18. Undifferentiated carcinoma, small cell type. This cancer is growing chiefly as sheets of small cells resembling lymphocytes, but in a few foci follicular arrangement is definite. (Hematoxylin and eosin, × 130.)

careful examination of most tumors will demonstrate recognizable epithelial structures such as abortive follicles. The other variety of small cell carcinoma grows more diffusely and is composed of masses of cells often resembling lymphocytes, reticulum cells, or plasma cells. In fact, it may be impossible to distinguish such a tumor from a lymphoma. As has been emphasized many times, the only way of establishing the diagnosis of small cell carcinoma of the diffuse type is by finding recognizable epithelial structures, such as abortive follicles (Fig. 4-18). Silver stains to demonstrate reticulum patterns are of little assistance in making the differential diagnosis between small cell carcinoma and lymphoma, but electron microscopic studies may be helpful. Both types of small cell carcinoma occur mostly in older women. The tumors rapidly invade the adjacent thyroid and the adjacent neck structures and metastasize extensively both to cervical lymph nodes and to more distant organs. The compact type has a slightly better prognosis than the diffuse type, but in either event, the prognosis is poor. The tumors are often inoperable at the time of diagnosis because of local extension or metastases. While generally not very responsive either to external irradiation or to radioiodine therapy, some patients receive good palliation from such treatment. Death usually results from the local extension of the tumor.

The *giant* or *spindle cell* carcinoma is the most malignant of the thyroid cancers and, indeed, is among the most malignant of all tumors of any location.[23] This is the one thyroid cancer in which there is often good suggestive evidence that its origin is either a benign adenoma or a differentiated carcinoma of long standing, as discussed elsewhere. Many patients give a history of a relatively stationary-sized mass in the neck for 10 or 15 years before the sudden onset of rapid growth, which is followed by death within a few months from giant cell carcinoma. Sometimes the outline of the circumscribed, partly calcified nodule may be identified within or adjacent to the giant cell cancer. Macroscopically the tumor is firm and almost always adherent to adjacent structures, so that resection in a curative sense is seldom possible. Histologically the tumor shows a massive overgrowth of spindle cells or giant cells or both with bizarre nuclei (Fig. 4–19). Mitoses, often atypical, are frequent. The microscopic appearance again resembles sarcoma more than carcinoma, and recognizable epithelial structures, while usually found, may be infrequent. Although lymph node and visceral metastases are common, the growth rate of the tumor is such that death from local extension occurs before metastases become very prominent. The prognosis is extremely poor, with only an occasional patient treated successfully.

Secondary Carcinoma

Tumor metastatic to the thyroid is relatively common. Silverberg and Vidone[45] found an incidence of 24 percent in 62 metastasizing cancers. The common tumors metastatic to the gland are those spreading by blood stream, such as carcinomas of the breast, lung, or kidney, and malignant melanoma.[40] Secondary tumor in the thyroid occasionally is confused with a primary thyroid cancer since the gross appearance may be very similar. It should be remembered that any tumor of the thyroid found in a patient who has or who has had cancer elsewhere capable of metastasis should be viewed with a possibility of its being a secondary tumor. As summarized by Elliott and Frantz,[8] many varieties of secondary tumors may present as a primary in the lung, breast, kidney, colon, and so forth, and all have metastasized to the thyroid where they have been mistaken for primary tumors. The secondary tumors may appear quite similar to the primary thyroid cancers grossly, although microscopically they usually are easily distinguished. The one exception is the renal cell carcinoma which, when metastatic to the thyroid, may look histologically very much like primary clear cell carcinoma of the thyroid.

SURGICAL PATHOLOGY

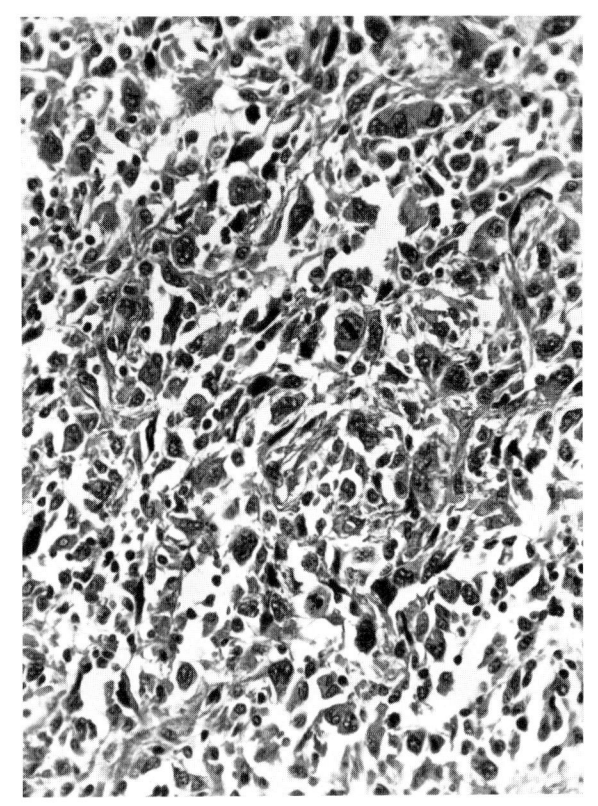

Figure 4–19. Undifferentiated carcinoma, giant cell type. This tumor is composed of bizarre giant cells and spindle cells and resembles sarcoma. Mitoses are frequent. Although the 70-year-old woman had had symptoms of hoarseness and cough for only one month, the tumor was fixed in the neck and had metastasized to the lungs. (Hematoxylin and eosin, × 130.)

Direct extension of adjacent carcinomas into the thyroid (for example, from carcinoma of the larynx) does occur, and most squamous cell carcinomas involving the thyroid represent such secondary extensions.

LYMPHOMA

Lymphoid tumors may involve the thyroid, either primarily or secondarily.[56] About 20 percent of patients with disseminated lymphoma show involvement of the thyroid at autopsy.[27] Primary lymphoma of the thyroid of various types also occurs but is rare and must be distinguished from small cell carcinoma as discussed elsewhere.

REFERENCES

1. Albores-Saavedra, J., Rose, G. G., Ibanez, M. L., et al.: The amyloid in solid carcinoma of the thyroid gland. Staining characteristics, tissue culture, and electron microscopic observations. Lab. Invest. 13:77–93 (Jan.) 1964.
2. Astwood, E. B.: Natural occurrence of antithyroid compounds as cause of simple goiter. Ann. Intern. Med. 30:1087–1103 (June) 1949
3. Carroll, R. E., Haddon, W., Jr., Handy, V. H., et al.: Thyroid cancer: Cohort analysis of increasing incidence in New York State, 1941–1962. J. Nat. Cancer Inst. 33:277–283 (Aug.) 1964
4. Catalona, W. J., Engelman, K., Ketcham, A. S., et al.: Familial medullary thyroid carcinoma, pheochromocytoma, and para-thyroid adenoma (Sipple's syndrome); study of a kindred. Cancer 28:1245–1254 (Nov.) 1971.
5. Conard, R. A., Rall, J. E., and Sutow, W. W.: Thyroid nodules as a late sequela of radioactive fallout, in a Marshall Island population exposed in 1954. New Eng. J. Med. 274:1391–1399 (June 23) 1966.
6. Cope, O., Rawson, R. W., and McArthur, J. W.: Hyperfunctioning single adenoma of thyroid. Surg. Gynec. Obstet. 84:415–426 (April) 1947.
7. Dube, W. J., Bell, G. O., and Aliapoulios, M. A.: Thyrocalcitonin activity in metastatic medullary thyroid carcinoma. Arch. Intern. Med. 123:423–427 (April) 1969.
8. Elliott, R. H., Jr., and Frantz, V. K.: Metastatic carcinoma masquerading as primary thyroid cancer: A report of authors' 14 cases. Ann. Surg. 151:551–561 (April) 1960.
9. Estimated cancer deaths and new cases by sex and site – 1971. *In* 1971 Cancer Facts and Figures. New York, American Cancer Society, Inc., 1970, p. 5.
10. Freeman, D., and Lindsay, S.: Medullary carcinoma of the thyroid gland. Arch. Path. 80:575–582 (Dec.) 1965.
11. Haber, M. H., and Lipkovic, P.: Thyroid cancer in Hawaii. Cancer 25:1224–1227 (May) 1970.
12. Hazard, J. B.: Thyroiditis: Review. Amer. J. Clin. Path. 25:289–298; 399–426 (March and April) 1955.
13. Hazard, J. B., Hawk, W. A., and Crile, G., Jr.: Medullary (solid) carcinoma of the thyroid; a clinicopathologic entity. J. Clin. Endocr. 19:152–161 (Jan.) 1959.
14. Hazard, J. B., and Kenyon, R.: Atypical adenoma of thyroid. Arch. Path. 58:554–563 (Dec.) 1954.
15. Hutter, R. V., Tollefsen, H. R., DeCosse, J. J., et al.: Spindle and giant cell metaplasia in papillary carcinoma of the thyroid. Amer. J. Surg. 110:660–668 (Oct.) 1965.
16. Ibanez, M. L., Russell, W. O., Albores-Saavedra, J., et al.: Thyroid carcinoma – biologic behavior and mortality. Postmortem findings in 42 cases, including 27 in which the disease was fatal. Cancer 19:1039–1052 (Aug.) 1966.
17. James, A. G.: Cancer Prognosis Manual. New York, American Cancer Society, Inc., 1966.
18. Kay, C., Abrahams, S., and McClain, P.: The weight of normal thyroid glands in children. Arch. Path. 82:349–352 (Oct.) 1966.
19. Klinck, G. H.: Structure of the thyroid. *In* Hazard, J. B., and Smith, D. E. (eds): The Thyroid. Baltimore, The Williams & Wilkins Co., 1964, pp. 1–31.
20. Klopp, C. T., and Kirson, S. M.: Therapeutic problems with ectopic non-cancerous follicular thyroid tissue in the neck: 18 case reports according to etiologic factors. Ann. Surg. 163:653–664 (May) 1966.
21. Long, R. T., Evans, A. M., and Beggs, J. H.: Surgical management of ectopic thyroid: Report of a case with simultaneous lingual and subhyoid median ectopic thyroid. Ann. Surg. 160:824–827 (Nov.) 1964.
22. Louw, J. H.: Congenital goitre. A review with a report of three cases of suffocative goitre in the newborn. S. Afr. Med. J. 37:976–983 (Sept. 28) 1963.
23. Meissner, W. A.: Undifferentiated carcinomas of the thyroid. International Union Against Cancer, Monograph Series 12. Berlin, Springer-Verlag, 1969, pp. 36–43.
24. Meissner, W. A., and Adler, A.: Papillary carcinoma of the thyroid; a study of the pathology of two hundred twenty-six cases. Arch. Path. 66:518–525 (Oct.) 1958.
25. Meissner, W. A., and Legg, M.A.: Persistent thyroid carcinoma. J. Clin. Endocr. 18:91–98 (Jan.) 1958.

26. Meissner, W. A., and McManus, R. G.: Comparison of histologic pattern of benign and malignant thyroid tumors. J. Clin. Endocr. 12:1474–1479 (Nov.) 1952.
27. Meissner, W. A., and Phillips, M. J.: Diffuse small-cell carcinoma of the thyroid. Arch. Path. 74:291–297 (Oct.) 1962
28. Meissner, W. A., and Warren, S.: Tumors of the thyroid gland. In Atlas of Tumor Pathology. 2nd series, fascicle 4. Washington, D. C., Armed Forces Institute of Pathology, 1969.
29. Melvin, K. E., Miller, H. H., Tashjian, A. H., Jr.: Early diagnosis of medullary carcinoma of the thyroid gland by means of calcitonin assay. New Eng. J. Med. 285:1115–1120 (Nov. 11) 1971.
30. Meyer, J. S., and Steinberg, L. S.: Microscopically benign thyroid follicles in cervical lymph nodes. Serial section study of lymph node inclusions and entire thyroid gland in 5 cases. Cancer 24:302–311 (Aug.) 1969.
31. Miller, J. M., Horn, R. C., and Block, M. A.: The evolution of toxic nodular goiter. Arch. Intern. Med. 113:72–88 (Jan.) 1964.
32. Mochizuki, Y., Mowafy, R., and Pasternack, B.: Weights of human thyroids in New York City. Health Phys. 9:1299–1301 (Dec.) 1963.
33. Patchefsky, A. S., Keller, I. B., and Mansfield, C. M.: Solitary vertebral column metastasis from occult sclerosing carcinoma of the thyroid gland: Report of a case. Amer. J. Clin. Path. 53:596–601 (May) 1970.
34. Pochin, E. E.: Prospects from the treatment of thyroid carcinoma with radioiodine. Clin. Radiol. 18:113–125 (April) 1967.
35. Polliack, A., and Freund, U.: Mixed papillary and follicular carcinoma of the thyroid gland with stromal amyloid. Amer. J. Clin. Path. 53:592–595 (May) 1970.
36. Pollock, W. F., and Stevenson, E. O.: Cysts and sinuses of the thyroglossal duct. Amer. J. Surg. 112:225–232 (Aug.) 1966.
37. Roth, S. I., Olen, E., and Hansen, L. S.: The eosinophilic cells of the parathyroid (oxyphil cells), salivary (oncocytes), and thyroid (Hürthle cells) glands. Light and electron microscopic observations. Lab. Invest. 11:933–941 (Nov.) 1962.
38. Sampson, R. J., Key, C. R., Buncher, C. R., et al.: Thyroid carcinoma in Hiroshima and Nagasaki. I. Prevalence of thyroid carcinoma at autopsy. J.A.M.A. 209:65–70 (July 7) 1969.
39. Sampson, R. J., Oka, H., Key, C. R., et al.: Metastases from occult thyroid carcinoma. An autopsy study from Hiroshima and Nagasaki, Japan. Cancer 25:803–811 (April) 1970.
40. Shimaoka, K., Takeuchi, S., and Pickren, J. W.: Carcinoma of thyroid associated with other primary malignant tumors. Cancer 20:1000–1005 (June) 1967.
41. Silberman, R., and Mendelson, I. R.: Teratoma of the neck; report of two cases and review of the literature. Arch. Dis. Child. 35:159–170 (April) 1960.
42. Silliphant, W. M., Klinck, G. H., and Levitin, M. S.: Thyroid carcinoma and death. A clinicopathological study of 193 autopsies. Cancer 17:513–525 (April) 1964.
43. Silverberg, S. G., Hutter, R. V., and Foote, F. W., Jr.: Fatal carcinoma of the thyroid: Histology, metastases, and causes of death. Cancer 25:792–802 (April) 1970.
44. Silverberg, S. G., and Vidone, R. A.: Carcinoma of the thyroid in surgical and postmortem material. Analysis of 300 cases at autopsy and literature review. Ann. Surg. 164:291–299 (Aug.) 1966a.
45. Silverberg, S. G., and Vidone, R. A.: Metastatic tumors in the thyroid. Pacif. Med. Surg. 74:175–180 (July–Aug.) 1966b.
46. Sinha, D., Pascal, R., and Furth, J.: Transplantable thyroid carcinoma induced by thyrotropin: Its similarity to human Hürthle cell tumors. Arch. Path. 79:192–198 (Feb.) 1965.
47. Stanbury, J. B.: Familial goiter. In Stanbury, J. B., Wyngaarden, J. B., and Fredrickson, D. S. (eds.): The Metabolic Basis of Inherited Disease. 2nd ed. New York, The Blakiston Division, McGraw-Hill Book Co., Inc., 1966, pp. 215–257.
48. Studer, H., and Greer, M. A.: A study of the mechanism involved in the production of iodine-deficiency goiter. Acta Endocr. 49:610–628 (Aug.) 1965.
49. Tollefsen, H. R., DeCosse, J. J., and Hutter, R. V.: Papillary carcinoma of the thyroid. A clinical and pathological study of 70 fatal cases. Cancer 17:1035–1044 (Aug.) 1964.
50. Welch, C. E.: Therapy for multinodular goiter. J.A.M.A. 195:339–341 (Jan. 31) 1966.
51. Williams, E. D., Brown, C. L., and Doniach, I.: Pathological and clinical findings in a

series of 67 cases of medullary carcinoma of the thyroid. J. Clin. Path. 19:103–113 (March) 1966.
52. Winship, T., and Rosvoll, R. V.: Childhood thyroid carcinoma. Cancer 14:734–743 (July-Aug.) 1961.
53. Woolner, L. B.: Thyroiditis: Classification and clinicopathologic correlation. *In* Hazard, J. B., and Smith, D. E. (eds.): The Thyroid. Baltimore, The Williams & Wilkins Co., 1964, pp. 123–142.
54. Woolner, L. B., Beahrs, O. H., Black, B. M., et al.: Classification and prognosis of thyroid carcinoma. A study of 885 cases observed in a thirty year period. Amer. J. Surg. 102:354–387 (Sept.) 1961.
55. Woolner, L. B., McConahey, W. M., and Beahrs, O. H.: Invasive fibrous thyroiditis (Riedel's struma). J. Clin. Endocr. 17:201–220 (Feb.) 1957.
56. Woolner, L. B., McConahey, W. M., Beahrs, O. H., et al.: Primary malignant lymphoma of the thyroid. Review of forty-six cases. Amer. J. Surg. 111:502–523 (April) 1966.

Chapter Five

THYROID PHYSIOLOGY AND FUNCTIONAL TESTS

Henry E. Zellmann, M.D.

The attention of surgeons, physicians, patients, and their families is often directed to the thyroid gland, to its function, and to its diagnostic tests. Most thyroid diseases respond favorably to treatment, and both patient and the medical team seek a cure.

By its anatomical position in the neck, the thyroid gland begs for attention. It is noteworthy for its accessibility to palpation, direct isotope measurement, and surgical attack. Had it evolved somewhere in the region of the pancreas, certainly much less would be made of it.

Since a high incidence of disease of the thyroid, certain psychophysiological syndromes such as globus hystericus and carotodynia, exposure of the neck to widespread inspection, a tendency to states of fatigue, anxiety, and depression, and obesity and fluid retention all have their common denominator in that they occur so often in women, it is no wonder that they comprise most of the thyroidologists' patients.

The thyroidologist spends much of his time defending the innocent thyroid gland from blame as the cause of psychoses, neuroses, situational reactions, obesity, and its opposite, anorexia nervosa. As the thyroid's advocate, he must frequently point the finger of guilt at the patient, her family, and occasionally her genes. To paraphrase Shakespeare, the fault lies not so much in her glands but in her "knives, forks, and spoons." On the other side of the coin, it is certainly true that thyroid disease may be so subtle as to go unnoticed, resulting in masked and apathetic hyperthyroidism. Thyroid hypofunction can also be hidden in such disguises as bizarre neurological, psychiatric, hematological, and rheumatoid syndromes.

IODIDE CYCLE

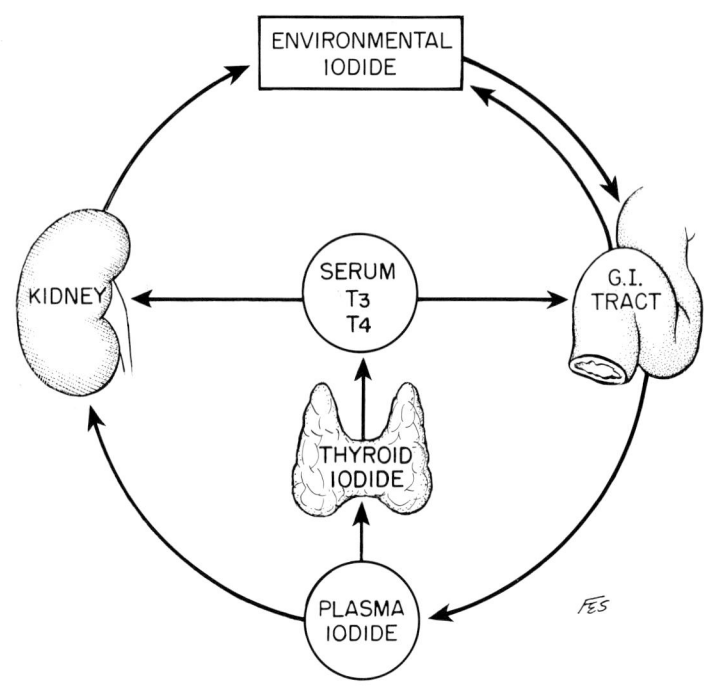

Figure 5-1. Iodide cycle.

THYROID PHYSIOLOGY

Although it would be beyond the scope of this chapter to attempt a full review, it is important that the surgeon be reasonably familiar with thyroid physiology, upon which functional tests are based. His colleague, the internist, is at times doubtful or in error, and certain laboratory results may be equivocal or occasionally in error; the patient may be pregnant or have used estrogens or iodides, and yet the surgeon must proceed. His treatments are often irrevocable and he must face the patient, the family, the tissue committee, and most importantly himself. What must he know? Briefly outlined, thyroid physiology involves the concentration of iodide with the production, storage, release, and fate of thyroid hormones.

Iodine and iodate are reduced in the process of digestion and circulate in the plasma as iodide (Fig. 5-1). Areas of concentration include the salivary and gastric glands but chiefly, of course, the thyroid gland. A high thyroid-plasma gradient exists, reaching, in Graves' disease 500 to 1. Iodide is oxidized probably by a peroxidase enzyme to iodine, which is bound to tyrosine in thyroglobulin to form either monoiodotyrosine (MIT) or diiodotyrosine (DIT) (Fig. 5-2). Coupling

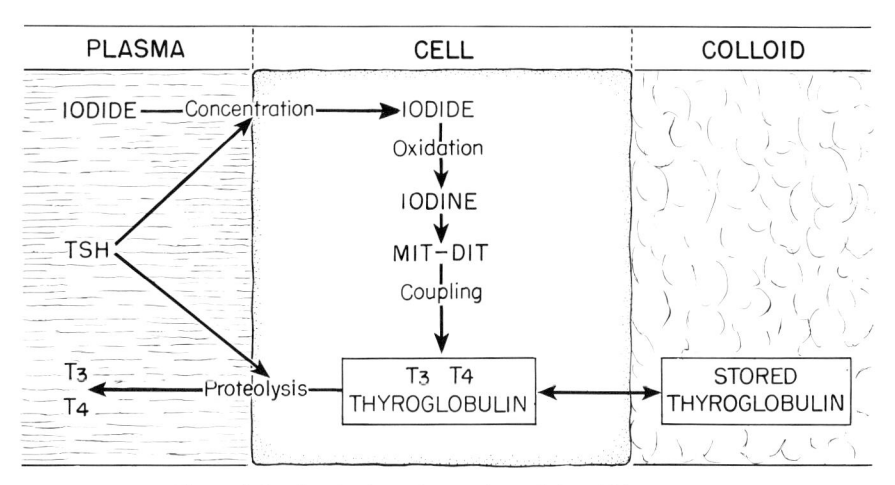

```
     PLASMA         |         CELL          |       COLLOID
  IODIDE —Concentration—→ IODIDE
                              ↓ Oxidation
                           IODINE
                              ↓
   TSH                     MIT–DIT
                              ↓ Coupling
                              ↓
    T3                    ┌─────────────┐      ┌──────────────┐
       ←—Proteolysis——    │   T3  T4    │ ←——→ │    STORED    │
    T4                    │THYROGLOBULIN│      │THYROGLOBULIN │
                          └─────────────┘      └──────────────┘
```

Figure 5–2. Synthesis and secretion of thyroid hormones.

by an appropriate enzyme produces either thyroxine (T4) or triiodothyronine (T3). Release of hormones stored in thyroglobulin is mediated by a proteolytic enzyme. These steps of synthesis and secretion are finely controlled by way of the hypothalamic-pituitary-thyroid feedback system (Fig. 5–3).

Alterations in the levels of free-circulating thyroid hormones influence the secretion of hypothalamic, thyrotropin-releasing hormone (TRH) which, through hypophyseal portal vessels, effects the release of thyrotropin-stimulating hormone (TSH). Kinetic studies show that, normally, approximately 90 μg. of T4 and 27 μg. of T3 are produced daily. Two thirds of the T3 is secreted by the thyroid gland and one third results from deiodination of T4 in vivo. It is likely then that T4 is a prohormone and that T3 plays the chief metabolic role.

Transport through the blood stream is by way of carriers, the serum proteins—specifically, thyroxine-binding globulin (TBG) and thyroxine-binding prealbumin (TBPA)—to sites of peripheral action where there is transfer, presumably to tissue TBG.

Plasma contains approximately 4 to 11 μg. of T4 and 0.1 to 0.2 μg. of T3 per 100 ml. Of these amounts, 0.05 percent of the former and 0.5 percent of the latter respectively are unbound. As can be seen, a higher percentage of T3 than T4 is free. Since T3 is three to four times more potent, its part in the metabolic equation is equal to that of T4.

MECHANISM OF ACTION OF T4 AND T3

T4 and T3 were identified 58 and 20 years ago respectively. We know they play a role in growth-energy metabolism, but it is surprising

PHYSIOLOGIC LEVEL OF THYROID FUNCTION TESTS

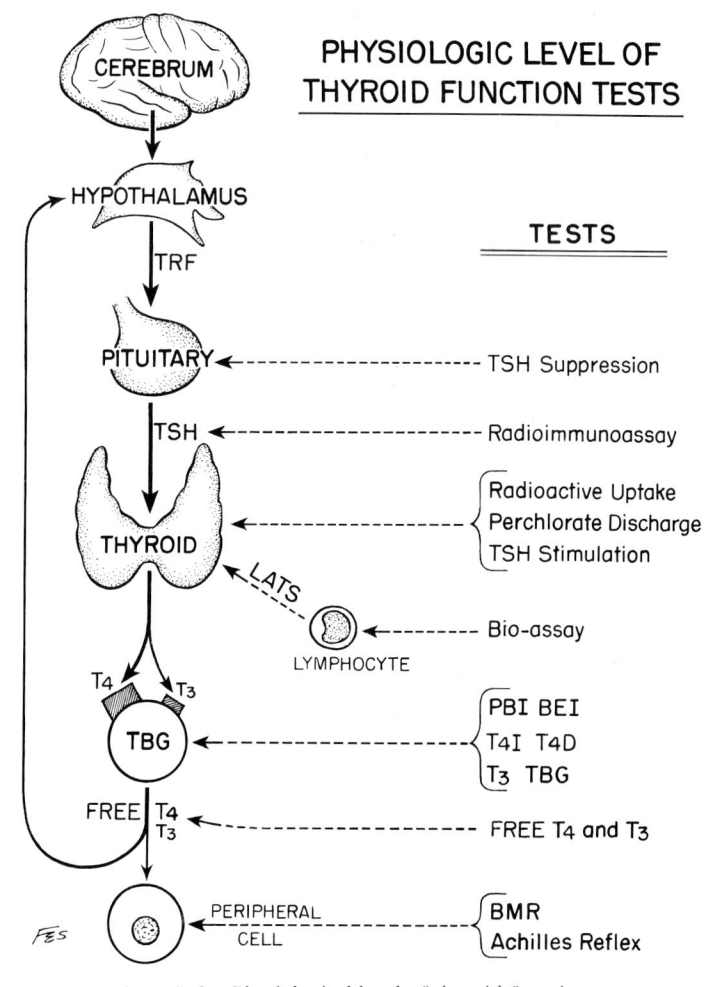

Figure 5-3. Physiological level of thyroid function tests.

that their precise mechanism of action still eludes us. A few facts have emerged: these hormones influence a wide variety of enzyme systems; their locus of action is on the mitochondrial membrane; oxidative phosphorylation is stimulated; and RNA polymerase succinoxidase, cytochromeoxidase, and adenosine triphosphatase are activated. The final common pathway of thyroid hormonal action may be its influence on protein synthesis, since this is an oxygen-dependent process. Such agents as puromycin, which inhibit protein synthesis, antagonize the action of T4.

Instead of a series of loosely related processes, we should try to view thyroid physiology as a fabric or framework on which we can place the patient, the illness, and the drugs or other agents which play their roles. Interestingly enough, most thyroid disease can be fitted nicely into such a scheme. Disorders of function may strike almost any part of this usually smooth-working system of supply and demand to produce clinical disease, with, as a rule, significant alteration in tests of thyroid activity.

THYROID FUNCTION TESTS

There has been a proliferation of laboratory tests of thyroid function from an era of relative famine to the present time of plenty. At one time a few primitive tests were available to study persons who, after investigation with the careful history and meticulous physical examination characteristic of the late 1800's and early 1900's, were suspected of having thyroid disease. Changes in quality, quantity, and delivery of medical care now require a variety of laboratory tests that frequently include assessment of thyroid function. At present, and certainly increasingly in the future, large populations will be evaluated. The yield of disease will be small, but the numbers of borderline results, laboratory errors, and nonthyroidal factors will be great.

A new dimension, then, has been added to clinical and laboratory medicine; that is, we now have a concept of examining the well or presumably well, where once we studied only the sick to find out what made them so and to estimate the extent and severity of their disease. Now we are examining millions of ostensibly healthy persons to detect a disease in its early stages when it is hopefully easier to cure or to control.

The clinician must keep in mind that automatic analyzers sometimes sacrifice precision for their tremendous variety in breadth and speed. They call attention to abnormal results which should stimulate more detailed history and physical examination and retesting along appropriate lines. Such multiphasic screening tests will identify, it is true, a few persons with unrecognized thyroid dysfunction, but for every such patient it is safe to say that thousands of abnormal tests will be found related to exogenous iodides or iatrogenic disturbances of TBG. It does not stretch the imagination too much to envision that, in the millennium which is presumably at hand, physicians will be dealing with a well tested automated society. The serum of most adults will be contaminated with radiographic iodide from semi-annual genitourinary and gastrointestinal surveys, women of child-bearing age will either be pregnant or possibly be taking oral contraceptives, and postmenopausal and menopausal women may be taking estrogens—all of which affect thyroid function tests.

Until the middle 1940's the life of the thyroidologist was relatively simple. He had only to learn the refinements of history taking and physical examination in a thyroid clinic and, when in doubt, resort to such simple measurements as were available to him—the basal metabolic rate and serum cholesterol. He was judge and jury. The evidence was elementary: to use iodide, to use thyroid substance, to operate, or not to operate. There followed an explosion of scientific information, perhaps loudest heard in the field of thyroid function tests; in fact, the reverberations are still being heard. The discovery of the radioactive isotopes of iodine, progress in electrophoresis of serum proteins, and radioimmunoassay have opened new avenues for physiological study and vastly complicated clinical testing and therapy. These advances have proved to be a mixed blessing.

Paradoxically, decision making, which should become easier and more accurate with the more information that is available, is, in fact, sometimes less easy and correct with a surfeit of tests. Another hazard of progress in thyroidology has been the rapidity with which new tests have evolved. It is probably no exaggeration to say that just when the personnel in the clinical and radioisotope laboratories become familiar with a technique, define its normal ranges and confidence limits, and achieve a high degree of sensitivity, and when the clinician becomes accustomed to this new test and applies it to a few of his patients, a new test appears! This is not to say that we are not grateful for these achievements. Fortunately the outlook now is not nearly so bleak, since many of these procedures have been relegated properly to physiological study.

The clinician must be familiar enough with past thyroid tests to judge a patient's history and to interpret retrospective studies, to be aware of the present available tests, their advantages and shortcomings, and at the same time to be flexible enough to yield to a truly better technique. In this day of changing values in so many spheres, it is no wonder that the physician and surgeon search for a few landmarks of stability amid this virtual storm of thyroid and other functional laboratory tests. I wish this chapter were the answer. Unfortunately it is less an answer than a guide to help the clinician judge today's patients with today's tests and to try to prepare him for tomorrow's patients and tomorrow's tests.

THYROID FUNCTION TESTS ON THE SERUM

Assessment of thyroid hormone levels by one or more serum tests[3, 7] is today the most widely used technique for several reasons: The patient is not required to visit the laboratory nor is he exposed to radiation; the specimens may be sent long distances for processing; and high levels of precision are achieved. There is usually a correlation between the magnitude of deviation from normal values and the severity of the illness. Serum tests are of two types: direct chemical measurement of iodide content, namely, protein-bound iodine (PBI), butanol-extractable iodide (BEI), and thyroxine iodide (T4I), and indirect tests involving estimates of thyroxine binding, namely, T3 and thyroxine displacement (T4D). Figure 5–3 presents a physiological view of thyroid function tests.

The PBI Test

The PBI test remains the most widely used laboratory estimate of thyroid activity and will likely maintain its position for several years. If the effects of pregnancy, estrogens, and iodides are taken into account, it is a very sensitive specific index with a range of 3.5 to 7.5 gamma per 100 ml.

It is wise to view all tests against a background of a bell curve of distribution to identify the few patients whose test results fall under the upper and lower limits of such curves. In this way we can account for the occasional patient who has a PBI of 2.5 and yet is perfectly normal from the endocrine standpoint and who has other causes of fatigue, change in weight, or other symptoms.

The PBI has the advantage of familiarity of long clinical and laboratory experience. Its shortcomings are well known. Since it measures extremely small amounts of iodide, contamination continues to be its chief drawback. Whereas at one time, in the absence of more specific treatments, iodides were a popular remedy, now therapy with iodides is limited almost exclusively to expectorants, dermatological, antihelminthic, and vitamin preparations. Diagnostically, however, the problem of organic iodides is great and will very likely increase. Inorganic iodide, although it reduces ^{131}I thyroidal uptake for several months, remains but a short time in the serum, interfering with the PBI determination no more than one or two weeks. Organic iodides, however, may have an effect on PBI levels for several months to a lifetime. The prime example of the latter is the cholecystographic dye, iophenoxic acid (Teridax), fortunately rarely used now, which elevates the PBI to levels of 1,000 to 2,000 gamma for many years or for life. Lymphangiographic agents should be placed in the same category. With modern cholecystographic dyes the PBI may be relied upon within 60 or fewer days, rarely longer. The PBI is also excellent for following response to therapy, with the exception that various thyroid hormones have differing effects, as indeed they have on other serum tests.

The BEI Test

The BEI test was devised to circumvent contamination by inorganic iodide, such as Lugol's solution and potassium iodide. It is normally 2 gamma less than the PBI. It is just as susceptible to organic iodide contamination, however, as the PBI. Technically a somewhat difficult procedure to carry out, the BEI test has been superseded by the T3 and T4D techniques.

The T3 Test

The T3 uptake test was discovered more or less by serendipity while Hamolsky and co-workers[2] were using radioactive T3 and T4 to study the peripheral activity of the thyroid hormones. Actually, the T3 test is an indirect estimate of the saturation of serum proteins, specifically TBG, with the patient's T4 and, to a lesser extent, T3. The technique employs a system in which a known amount of T3 labeled with ^{131}I seeks out the remaining binding sites on TBG and the excess binds to whatever competing tissue or other substance is available; hence, the high uptake in these areas in hyperthyroidism and the opposite in myxedema when sites on the patient's proteins are unsaturated and accept most of the labeled hormone. At the present time, ion exchange resin[8] is used, although the test was originally performed with red blood cells and, indeed, initial work showed that minced muscle and white blood cells also attracted T3. Its range is 25 to 35 percent, but there are several methods of expressing its result, namely, a ratio. The T3 is unaffected by any kind of iodide, organic or inorganic, since it is not this element that is being measured but rather the binding of it on the patient's serum proteins. Whatever influences T4-binding protein and thyroid hormone binding also influences T3, PBI, T4I, and T4D results. There may be congenital elevations or reductions in TBG or similar responses because of estrogens or androgens. Such drugs as salicylates and diphenylhydantoin interfere with binding of thyroid hormones to TBG.

The T4I Test

This procedure, which was conceived to eliminate iodide contamination which so plagued the PBI test, involves elution of T4 from serum by column resin chromatography. It is an excellent test with limits similar to the PBI: 3.5 to 6.5 gamma per 100 ml. It is not influenced by inorganic iodides in any way. Although it can signal the presence of an organic iodine in the specimen, it can go no further and, hence, is not yet the ideal test.

The T4D Test

The T4D is the best serum thyroid test presently available.[5] It is not influenced by iodides of any sort. It is a competition test somewhat similar to the T3, although more complex. A measured amount of TBG and a measured amount of T4 labeled with ^{125}I are added to the patient's serum, which has been deproteinized. In other words, all TBG has been destroyed and T4 has been completely freed. T4 attaches to the fixed amount of TBG, and the added labeled T4 fills in the remaining sites. Comparison with standard curves reveals the patient's levels of serum T4. There are at least two disadvantages to this test: anything affecting the serum TBG as well as any drugs influencing binding (salicylates, phenylbutazone, and so forth) will change its results, just as it will the PBI and T3. The other shortcoming, which time may solve as limits are more precisely defined, is that the "normal" range appears to be rather wide — 4 to 11 gamma — since it presumably measures the entire T4 molecule instead of the narrower limits of 3.5 to 7.5 for PBI and T4I.

As we can see, the chief shortcoming of the T4D and resin T3 (RT3) tests are related to disturbances of TBG. If both tests are carried out, we can identify these variations, but we are unable to estimate the patient's thyroid state in a quantitative way. Because of the reciprocal relationships of the RT3 on the one hand, and the T4D and PBI on the other, their product, termed the "free thyroxine index," does reflect the true thyroid status in a numerical fashion. The effective thyroxine ratio (ETR) is a promising single test assessing both TBG capacity and total serum T4.

Peripheral Function Tests

Our most serious deficiency in assessing thyroid function is the lack of an accurate index of hormonal action in the tissues. Theoretically the basal metabolic rate (BMR) and Achilles reflex are the only indexes of peripheral action of thyroid hormones. Realistically, however, they are very crude indicators, remote from the thyroid itself certainly, and it would seem also equally remote from the site of action of T3 and T4, which is in the subcellular and cellular levels where the metabolic action is.

BMR. It is fortunate that the resurgence of interest in the BMR has subsided. Reappraisal was attempted because clinicians were discouraged by the multiplicity of thyroid function tests and the many extrathyroid factors that were influencing them. While the BMR is unaffected by iodides or estrogens, it also seems insensitive to all but the most obvious changes in thyroid activity. It is now chiefly of historical interest.

Achilles Reflex. When the Achilles stretch reflex test appeared on the scene, it was hailed as being as unaffected by extrathyroid factors as was the BMR. It was the airless, bloodless, painless, most simple, and rapid of the available tests. All these features it no doubt had; unfortunately it also had outstanding shortcomings — it lacked sensitivity and specificity.

Since the Achilles reflex meter, like the BMR machine, is frequently a part of the physician's office equipment, having once been acquired it may be given up reluctantly. Now and then a clinician seems to make do with a BMR or Achilles reflex test; this is because he is an excellent clinician, not because of the accuracy of these tests.

RADIOACTIVE IODINE UPTAKE

Iodine-131 techniques are discussed in detail elsewhere in this volume and are mentioned here merely for comparison. Uptakes of ^{131}I at intervals after a tracer dose have their greatest usefulness in the diagnosis of Graves' disease and in judging the amount of ^{131}I needed for its therapy. They are of less value in myxedema unless clearly shown to be less than 5 to 10 percent in 24 hours.

Isotope scanning is useful for outlining hyperfunctioning and hypofunctioning nodules of various kinds, namely, neoplasm, thyroiditis, cyst, and adenomatous goiter. Nodules smaller than 2 cm. usually do not lend themselves to scanning.

When results of all serum and routine ^{131}I tests are borderline or equivocal, as does happen, the suppression test[1] with T3 may be decisive, since the hyperplastic gland of Graves' disease as well as the hyperfunctioning nodule are autonomous.

The thyroid response to exogenous TSH as measured by a rise in the uptake of ^{131}I or an elevation in serum thyroid tests, or both, is useful in differentiating primary from secondary myxedema. It is helpful also in assessing states of low thyroid reserve and in identifying patients who are unnecessarily taking thyroid substance.

The introduction of iodate in the making of bread has tended to lower "normal" ^{131}I uptake values.[6]

DISEASES OF THE THYROID

Against the background of these functional tests, let us see how diseases of the thyroid influence their values.

Iodide Lack. The classic endemic goiter is presumed to result from TSH stimulation of a thyroid struggling to make adequate hormone from an insufficient supply of iodide in the diet. The uptake of ^{131}I is usually elevated, whereas the serum level of T4 is either normal or low. Other less familiar causes of lack of iodide in nonendemic goiter areas are dietary faddism, chronic alcoholism, and vigorous diuresis.[4]

Iodide Excess. Although it is recognized that a normal diet should contain at least 50 μg. (ideally 150 to 200 μg.) of iodide daily, it is perhaps less well known that prolonged administration of large amounts of iodides of the order of 1,000 to 1,500 mg. a day may in itself induce goiter or myxedema or both.

Such iodide goiters occur during therapy of asthma, bronchitis, or emphysema in certain vulnerable individuals in whom the thyroid gland is unable to overcome the inhibitory effect of iodide on T4 production and release. Goiter is, then, a response to TSH stimulation. This sensitivity to iodides is a feature both of Hashimoto's and Graves' diseases and accounts for the moderate effectiveness of so simple a preparation as Lugol's solution in the therapy of the latter.

Disorders of Formation

The common sporadic nontoxic nodular goiter (adenomatous goiter) is very likely the result of a subtle fault in hormonogenesis in which, either intermittently or steadily, TSH must stimulate the thyroid beyond physiological limits to maintain the patient at a euthyroid level. At times a state of mild myxedema is the best that can be achieved. Although uncommon, certain genetically determined biochemical lesions may produce goiter and myxedema resulting from deficiencies of enzymes required in the several steps of thyroid hormone production. The most unusual of these lies in the trapping or concentrating mechanism. The most frequently observed enzyme disorder is in the next step, a peroxidase lack. Deficiencies of coupling and deiodinating enzymes are rare. The clinical pictures and laboratory results vary in degree, depending on the severity of the enzymic defect. Profound myxedema (goitrous cretinism) may be present from the outset, or the fault may be mild enough merely to produce goiter in an otherwise euthyroid state. Except in inborn errors of the trapping mechanism, ^{131}I uptakes because of TSH effect are often high. PBI values may be high also when abnormal iodoproteins are present which are noncalorigenic and yet contain iodides to be measured in a PBI test. Lack of deiodinating enzyme within the thyroid may produce a spillover of iodoproteins in the blood, and these may be recovered in the urine. Failure to oxidize iodides may result in adequate and even high initial uptake (trapping) of iodide but almost complete absence of organic binding to the thyronine molecule, so that trapped iodide may be displaced from the thyroid easily by perchlorate or other large anions such as thiocyanate. Since this anion competes with iodide for the iodide space, this technique, the perchlorate discharge test,[10] detects faulty organification of iodide.

The deceptive nature of these enzymic disorders can be appreciated when we realize that the patient may have a goiter, a high PBI, a high uptake of ^{131}I and, most surprisingly, primary hyperplasia, which may be present on pathologic examination, yet the patient may not have hypermetabolism. Fortunately the T4D, BEI, and the T4I tests measure accurately true calorigenic hormone, and great dissociation between PBI and these tests may suggest an enzymic fault. In other words, the serum T4D, T4I, and BEI are normal or low and the PBI is high. The proper treatment for such a goiter is thyroid substance — not thyroidectomy.

Quantitative Disorders

Diffuse Toxic Goiter. Graves' disease remains a mysterious syndrome in which the entire thyroid gland acts in an autonomous fashion. It is frequently explosive in onset, with no previous history of goiter. Although severity varies considerably, all or most of the serum functional tests are elevated; an uptake of ^{131}I is high in three hours and the 24-hour uptake exceeds 40 percent. The hallmark of Graves' disease, from the laboratory standpoint, is the inability to suppress whatever uptake is found with 100 μg. of T3 or its equivalent in other thyroid substance within a week or more of therapy. The normal thyroid ^{131}I uptake is suppressed by at least 50 percent by this dose.

Nodular Toxic Goiter. It is well known that the clinical pattern of Plummer's disease may be obscure. Unfortunately the laboratory data may often be just as inconclusive. It is a disease notorious for borderline or normal serum test. Twenty-four-hour uptakes of ^{131}I are normal in 50 to 70 percent of patients with toxic nodular goiter. The radioactive scintiscan is one of the most helpful laboratory tests, since usually one and occasionally more hyperfunctioning areas can be found. Hyperfunctioning nodules are usually 2.5 to 3 cm. or more in diameter.

Just as the distribution of laboratory tests is varied, clinical manifestations both of Graves' disease and Plummer's disease form a spectrum, a kaleidoscopic pattern. Plummer's disease begins in a gradual, most subtle manner since it is an event in the natural history of nodular goiter which often has a span of 20 to 40 years or more before reaching a state of hypermetabolism. With the present trend toward surgical restraint in dealing with persons with nodular goiter, it is possible to observe a rise in serum thyroid tests from normal to hyperthyroid levels occurring over a period of several years to the point of hypermetabolism. The level of clinical toxicity is reached so slowly that, since it usually occurs in persons aged 60 to 70 years and more often when disabilities in the cardiovascular system are common, it may easily be overlooked. Graves' disease, on the other hand, is a vigorous process, from the laboratory as well as from the clinical standpoint.

T3 Thyrotoxicosis. When the PBI tests were first used, clinicians recognized that occasionally a patient who presented with overwhelming clinical evidence of hyperthyroidism, yet had serum levels of thyroid hormone that were completely normal. They responded to antithyroid therapy in the usual fashion, and it was found that their thyroid glands were autonomous, usually nodular, and nonsuppressible by exogenous thyroid substance. The details of this entity gradually became clearer as methods were devised to measure precisely serum levels of T3.[3]

Hashimoto's Thyroiditis. Tests for this disease vary tremendously, depending on the stage at which the "laboratory biopsy" is made. The PBI may be elevated early in its course because inefficient thyroid cells are responding to TSH stimulation by producing, as best they can, iodinated protein measurable by the PBI technique but not always conforming to the classic T3 and T4 configuration. Here again, as in some congenital hyperplastic goiters, the serum tests which measure most closely the true T3 and T4 values—BEI, serum T4, and T4I—are accurate. A significant dissociation between these tests and the PBI is a clue to the Hashimoto process. This combination of a high PBI and ^{131}I uptake may be very puzzling to the clinician in some of the early stages of Hashimoto's disease when there may be signs and symptoms of hypermetabolism.

The laboratory and clinical pictures at times mimic Graves' disease.

Additional help from the laboratory may be obtained by both simple and complex procedures. The simple procedures are an elevated erythrocyte sedimentation rate (ESR) and the protein flocculation tests such as thymol turbidity, which may reach levels of 40 or more units in the absence of liver disease. However, more specific tests detecting thyroid autoantibodies are available.

At the other end of the spectrum of Hashimoto's process is exhaustion of thyroid function with low serum thyroid tests and a low ^{131}I uptake. In fact, spontaneous myxedema is viewed as a variant of chronic thyroiditis in which there is more destruction and atrophy rather than exuberant lymphocytic and fibroblastic proliferation and enlargement.

Subacute Thyroiditis. This is a disorder similar to Hashimoto's thyroiditis in which the timing of laboratory testing is crucial to proper interpretation of results. Initially the serum tests (the PBI, T3 and T4D) are almost always elevated, whereas ^{131}I uptakes are extremely low, 0 to 1 or 2 percent. A mild normocytic and normochromic anemia may be present, and a markedly elevated ESR, often in the range of 100 mm. or more an hour, is typical. With resolution of the process, functional tests return to normal levels. Permanent myxedema should not occur. Indeed, few documented cases have been reported, and these have followed several attacks of thyroiditis. Confusion can occur in a patient who had been made hypermetabolic by the liberation of two or more months' supply of thyroid hormone within a week or two, who shows peripheral signs of hypermetabolism, and who has elevated serum thyroid tests and a goiter more or less tender (occasionally the gland in Graves' disease is tender). A low ^{131}I uptake should establish the diagnosis of subacute thyroiditis.

Malignant Exophthalmos and the Long-acting Thyroid Stimulator (LATS). To his dismay, the thyroid surgeon occasionally observes that a patient he had most carefully prepared for operation, on whom he had skillfully performed subtotal thyroidectomy and who had been restored to a perfectly euthyroid state, proceeds to the development of the dreaded complication of Graves' disease—malignant exophthalmos. An understanding of the natural history of this process will help to relieve any feeling of guilt and reassure the patient of the surgeon's blamelessness in what might prove to be a very unpleasant outcome. It is best to view Graves' disease as a syndrome having two possible components: one of hypermetabolism with or without diffuse goiter (since 2 percent of patients have no demonstrable goiter), and one of an infiltrative dermal and ocular component. The latter may be mild, consisting of stare and lid lag with or without proptosis, or may be severe, described by various terms as endocrine, malignant, or progressive exophthalmos, and ranging from sensations of irritation to excessive lacrimation, chemosis, orbital edema, optic atrophy, disorders of extraocular muscle motility, inability to close the eyelids with resulting exposure keratitis, and corneal ulcer occasionally proceeding to panophthalmitis requiring enucleation. The disease may run its entire course with hypermetabolism as its only manifestation, or exophthalmos may be its single feature. The eye and thyroid components may coincide or one may precede the other by as long as 30 years, making short-term observations in this condition of little value.

Some time in the course of Graves' disease there can usually be detected in the serum an antibody of the 7S globulin type, LATS. Presumably it is produced in lymphoid tissue, probably as a response to an antigen in the thyroid cell, although this is still a controversial point. Previously it was thought to correspond very closely to the activity of progressive exophthalmos and to have its highest titer at that time, but now it is believed to be related more to the phase of hypermetabolism than to ophthalmopathy. When LATS was thought to have had a prominent etiologic role in this type of exophthalmos and that lowering the titer would be helpful, attempts were made to destroy every last thyroid cell by such enthusiastic measures as total thyroidectomy followed by ablation of any remnant of thyroid tissue, not only by ^{131}I but also by the stimulation of such remnants beforehand by TSH. At times the LATS test may be of value in differentiating severe exophthalmos occurring rarely in certain patients with orbital and periorbital tumors, Hashimoto's thyroiditis, Cushing's syndrome, and acromegaly, since LATS is uniformly absent in these diseases.

It is comforting to the surgeon and to his patients with progressive exophthalmos that the illness may either precede or follow not only surgical but also medical and radioactive treatment of hyperthyroidism or, indeed, no treatment whatsoever.

THYROACTIVE DRUGS

In properly interpreting results of the several thyroid function tests performed on serum, the surgeon must know the type of thyroactive drugs his patient is using as replacement therapy. Desiccated thyroid contains both L-thyroxine and L-triiodothyronine and, in the customary doses of 120 to 180 mg. daily, it tends to produce physiological levels of PBI and other serum tests, T3, T4D, and T4I. Certain lots of thyroglobulin, since they contained less T4 in proportion than desiccated thyroid, yielded, at least previously, a lower PBI since T3 is not measured. Full doses of triiodothyronine sodium liothyronine (Cytomel), namely, 50 to 100 μg. daily for the same reason, lower all serum thyroid tests, although the patient remains completely euthyroid. Synthetic thyroxine (Synthroid or Letter), on the other hand, is tightly bound to TBG and produces elevated serum tests in persons who feel perfectly fit from the thyroid standpoint. Synthetic thyroid substances such as liotrix (Euthroid, Thyrolar) containing a physiological balance of T4:T3 in a ratio of 4:1 are now available.

PREOPERATIVE EVALUATION

The surgeon must always be alert for the person desiring elective or other surgical procedures who has no obvious clinical thyroid dysfunction but who has mild myxedema or hyperthyroidism. Operations on either type of patient can be disastrous. On the one hand, persons with myxedema are exquisitely sensitive to many drugs, cardiac and respiratory arrest, intestinal and bladder atony, and difficulty with aspiration of bronchial secretions; yet, on the other hand, it is well known how the stress of anesthesia and surgery, however slight, evokes a thyroid storm in persons with what appears to be the mildest hyperthyroidism. There is no precise relationship between the level of serum tests and the probability of storm.

THYROCALCITONIN

The importance of calcitonin in calcium homeostasis in normal man is uncertain. It may play its role only during the fetal life as a developmental hormone. It is produced in the parafollicular cells of the thyroid gland. Its measurement in the serum is uniquely helpful in detecting clinically inapparent medullary carcinoma of the thyroid. Its presence in relatives of patients who have the syndrome of bilateral pheochromocytoma, perioral mucosal neuromas, and medullary carcinoma of the thyroid justifies prophylactic thyroidectomy. Recurrence of primary medullary carcinoma as well as metastatic foci usually causes elevated serum calcitonin levels. Surprisingly, hypocalcemia is uncommon and is usually accompanied by levels of calcitonin 1,000 to 2,000 times normal. Medullary carcinoma commonly elevates calcitonin 100 times normal.

SUMMARY

Frequently the diagnosis of thyroid dysfunction is clear at a glance. At times, one or more laboratory tests are needed. Occasionally the answer may elude even the most sophisticated studies, necessitating either observation and retesting after the passage of time or a trial of medical therapy. We should learn to use restraint before committing the patient to destructive therapy, either surgical or radioiodine.

We must recognize the inherent, almost infinite, biologic variability of the patients, with their wide range of differences, whether in heights, weights, personality structure, or PBI. For this reason it is unrealistic to expect our laboratories to devise a single test with normal and pathologic limits so sharply defined that there is absolutely no overlap. What the physician and surgeon do expect perhaps is two tests which will yield 90 to 95 percent precision and which, when combined with clinical experience, the history, and physical examination, should result in diagnostic accuracy approaching 98 to 100 percent.

The ultimate single serum thyroid function test would theoretically be the serum-free T4, since it is this level which determines sickness or health from the thyroid standpoint. It is far from the ideal single test because it requires that either a valid PBI be possible, excluding all patients who have had iodide contamination in their serum, or that a serum T4D be available. The determination of free T4 is technically not a simple procedure, and the amount measured is so small (millimicrograms) that it would seem that the possibility of error would be high. Free T3 is even more difficult to measure.

At the present time the minimum screening for thyroid function would be a PBI. Clearly abnormal and borderline results call for a clinical review of the patient, a repetition of the PBI to eliminate technical error, and usually a battery of T3 and T4D. The latter two tests are reciprocally affected by the estrogens and androgens as well as inherited disorders of TBG.

To eliminate retesting, an initial screen might include either a PBI or T4D combined with a T3 test. If the levels of T3, T4D, and PBI are elevated, hyperthyroidism is almost invariably present. The reverse usually means hypothyroidism. Elevated PBI and T4 and low T3 indicate either estrogen excess or congenital increase in TBG; depressed PBI and T4 and elevated T3 mean either androgen excess or diminished TBG. Great dissociation between PBI and T4D levels, namely, significantly higher PBI than T4D, is consistent with enzyme-deficient goiter or Hashimoto's thyroiditis, in which noncalorigenic fragments of the iodothyronines are present in the serum.

The new ETR may someday be the most useful single serum test.

REFERENCES

1. Greer, M. A., and Smith, G. E.: Method for increasing accuracy of radioiodine uptake as test for thyroid function by use of desiccated thyroid. J. Clin. Endocr. 14:1374–1384 (Nov.) 1954.
2. Hamolsky, M. W., Stein, M., and Freedberg, A. S.: The thyroid hormone-plasma protein complex in man. II. A new in vitro method for study of uptake of labelled hormonal components by human erythrocyte. J. Clin. Endocr. 17:33–43 (Jan.) 1957.
3. Handbook of Specialized Diagnostic Laboratory Tests. 8th ed. Van Nuys, California, Bio-Science Latoratories, October, 1968.
4. Mehbod, H., Swartz, C. D., and Brest, A. N.: The effect of prolonged thiazide administration on thyroid function. Arch. Intern. Med. 119:283–286 (March) 1967.
5. Murphy, B. E., and Pattee, C. J.: Determination of thyroxine utilizing the property of protein-binding. J. Clin. Endocr. 24:187–196 (Feb.) 1964.
6. Pittman, J. A., Jr., Daily, G. E., 3d, and Beschi, R. J.: Changing normal values for thyroidal radioiodine uptake. New Eng. J. Med. 280:1431–1434 (June 26) 1969.
7. Selenkow, H. A., and Refetoff, S.: Common tests of thyroid function in serum. J.A.M.A. 202:135–136 (Oct. 9) 1967.
8. Sterling, K., and Tabachnick, M.: Resin uptake of I-131 triiodothyronine as a test of thyroid function. J. Clin. Endocr. 21:456–464 (April) 1961.
9. Sterling, K., Bellabarba, D., Newman, E. S., et al.: Determination of triiodothyronine concentration in human serum. J. Clin. Invest. 48:1150–1158 (June) 1969.
10. Stewart, R. D., and Murray, I. P.: An evaluation of the perchlorate discharge test. J. Clin. Endocr. 26:1050–1058 (Oct.) 1966.

Chapter Six

THE SURGICAL SIGNIFICANCE OF THYROID ISOTOPOLOGY: MORPHOLOGIC AND PHYSIOLOGIC CONSIDERATIONS

Ferris J. Siber, M.D.

The delineation of an organ by radioisotopic scanning (rectilinear or camera techniques) depends on the selective concentration or retention of the radiopharmaceutical tracer by that organ. In 1951 Cassen and his associates[15] described techniques for thyroid imaging using radioactive iodine (^{131}I) and a moving mechanical detector, that is, automatic radioisotope scanning. Previously investigators had relied upon manual detectors (collimated Geiger counters) to obtain counts over segments of the thyroid gland in order to determine the presence or absence of "hot" or "cold" nodules. The isotopic technique of depicting the thyroid gland depends on the avidity of the thyroid tissue for iodine. This procedure provides information regarding the position, size, and shape of the gland and allows the assessment of nodular areas of either increased or decreased isotopic localization.[42]

Thyroid scanography[12] is of great value in the following instances:

1. Outlining nodules and determining their status ("hot," "warm," "cool," or "cold").

2. Evaluating chronic thyroiditis, lobulations, and asymmetry of the gland.

3. Detecting intrathoracic extension of thyroid tissue.
4. Identifying masses in the neck or mediastinum as being of thyroidal or nonthyroidal origin.
5. Evaluating the patient with carcinoma of the thyroid before and after ablation of the gland for the identification of pulmonary and other metastatic lesions.
6. Examining a patient after various types of thyroid resections. It is common to detect a significant amount of thyroid tissue left intact to preserve the parathyroid glands.

INSTRUMENTATION

The two classes of radiation detectors commercially available are the moving rectilinear scanner with a focusing collimator and the stationary, rapid-imaging gamma camera.

The Rectilinear Scanner

In the rectilinear scanner the detecting probe usually contains a thallium-activated sodium iodide crystal with a 5-inch, coarse-focus lead collimator. The detecting probe moves across (from right to left), down, and then across (from left to right) over the thyroidal area, with a spacing of 1 to 2 mm. between the scans (Fig.6–1). Therefore, the gland is imaged sequentially (rather than simultaneously as in the gamma camera).

The gamma rays emitted by the radionuclide within the thyroid gland are received by the detecting crystal after passing through a number of tapered holes in a lead block. This lead collimator is designed to allow only the gamma rays directly beneath the holes to reach the crystal and therefore attempts to exclude neighboring radiation.

By a complex system of energy conversions and electronic circuitry, the pattern of radioactivity is recorded photographically on unexposed x-ray film and mechanically on white paper. A maximum area of radio-

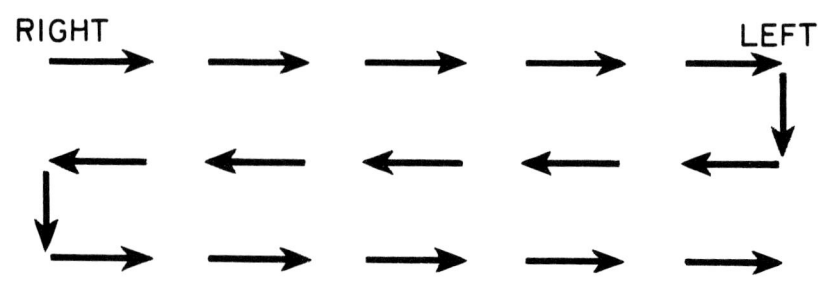

Figure 6–1. Pattern of probe movement across patient.

activity within the thyroid gland appears as an area of maximum blackening on the developed x-ray film or as a maximum number of dots on the paper.

The Gamma Camera

The gamma camera is an electronic device capable of recording the distribution of radioactivity within an organ.[3-5, 17, 57] This rapid-imaging system utilizes electronic circuitry to produce flashes on an oscilloscope. The actual organ image (scintigram) is obtained by recording the flashes on the oscilloscope with a Polaroid camera. Therefore, the pattern of radioactivity is transmitted *simultaneously* from all points to the face of a stationary crystal, permitting rapid visualization of the radioactivity over the entire thyroidal area.[2, 29, 41]

RADIONUCLIDES UTILIZED IN SCANNING THE THYROID GLAND

The radionuclides currently available include ^{131}I (and to a lesser degree other isotopes of iodine), technetium (^{99m}TcO$_4^-$), and ^{75}Se-selenomethionine.

As is true in cases of other medications, the administration of radiopharmaceuticals to pregnant or lactating women or to patients under the age of 18 years requires careful evaluation by the physician. The use of any radioactive substance and its attendant acceptable radiation is justified only by the seriousness of the lesion under consideration.

Iodine

Physical Characteristics. Clinically, probably the most commonly used isotope of iodine is ^{131}I, which is derived from products of uranium fission or the neutron bombardment of tellurium. Iodine-131 has a physical half-life of 8.05 days. On disintegration it produces five major gamma rays: 0.364 Mev. (numerically this is the most important in that 82 percent of the gamma rays have this energy), 0.638 Mev., 0.284 Mev., 0.724 Mev., and 0.08 Mev. Also, on disintegration ^{131}I produces a beta particle with an average energy of 0.188 Mev. The final disintegration product is xenon-131.

The gamma rays have high penetrability and escape from the body. Therefore, the gamma emission can be detected by suitable crystals in an external detecting probe and thereby measured easily.

The short range of the beta particles in tissue (average, 0.5 mm., and maximum, 2 mm.) accounts for their almost complete absorption within the thyroid tissue. They are responsible for 90 percent of the radiation dose to the gland and therefore for the biological action of iodine-131.

Other isotopes of iodine such as ^{125}I and ^{123}I, which have different physical half-lives and radiation characteristics, have also been used in clinical isotopology.[16, 43]

Approximately 24 hours before scanning, a capsule containing a tracer dose of 20 to 40 microcuries (μCi.) of sodium radioactive iodide (^{131}I) is administered orally. (We administer 1,000 μCi. if pulmonary or other metastases are to be detected.)

The sodium radioiodide (^{131}I) is tightly absorbed on the inner walls of the gelatin capsule. Therefore, the capsule contains nothing that can be spilled.

Frontal Scan. The thyroid area is examined with the patient in the supine position. The detecting probe moves in a caudad direction toward the suprasternal notch and down to the thorax if intrathoracic extension is to be confirmed. A suspicious area may be reexamined with the patient in the right or left lateral position.

The gamma ray spectrometer has been peaked to accept the specific gamma energy of iodine-131, with the lower and upper window settings at 335 to 395 kev., respectively. The technical factors are as follows: 5-inch by 2-inch thallium-activated sodium iodide crystals; 14-inch by 17-inch x-ray film with small light source for photoscanning; white paper, 8-inch by 10-inch for dot scan; and dot factor, 4. The contrast range differential is determined by the difference between the maximum and minimum counts per minute. Additional factors include a scan speed of 40 cm. per minute; density, 75; high voltage, 1,300; line spacing, 2 mm.; and background cut-off, 0 percent. Geographical marks are placed over the thyroid and the suprasternal notches.

Technetium

Technetium (^{99m}TcO$_4^-$) is a decay product of the parent molybdenum-99 (^{99}Mo) and is separated from the parent isotope by a relatively simple "milking" process. The molybdenum parent decays and generates technetium, which is then removed from the generating column by selective elution.[23, 46]

Physical Characteristics. Technetium has a physical half-life of six hours. On disintegration it produces gamma ray emission of 140 kev. and no beta radiation. This "clean" gamma emission and rapid rate of radioactive decay result in a minimal radiation dose to the patient and to the thyroid gland.

The pertechnetate is trapped by the thyroid gland in a manner similar to that of iodide, but unlike iodide it is not converted into organic forms and "leaks" out of the gland.[1, 7, 19] Therefore, there is only a minimal short-term radiation hazard. After the oral or intravenous administration of 1 to 2 mCi., the technetium is concentrated in the thyroid, salivary glands, stomach, colon, and urinary bladder.

Technetium is considered a satisfactory thyroid scanning agent when compared to ^{131}I for the following reasons: (1) A lower radiation dose is delivered to the patient because of the "clean" low energy of the gamma ray emission and short half-life. Also, the thyroid gland receives only about 0.001 of the radiation dose.[46] (2) Higher count rates are obtained over the thyroid because a larger tracer dose (1 or 2 mCi.) may be administered. Indeed, counting rates 10 to 25 times those of iodine can be obtained;[52] therefore, scanning time is significantly reduced. (3) The ability to administer large doses results in improved spatial resolution. (4) A more efficient collimation may be achieved because of the lower energy gamma radiation emitted. (5) Useful scans may be obtained in patients with hypothyroidism and also when radioactive iodide uptake has been suppressed by exogenous iodide, thyroid hormone, or antithyroid drugs.[54] Scanning with pertechnetate is useful in patients with diminished accumulation of radioactive iodine because the larger doses of technetium provide better visualization of the gland. (6) A scan revealing useful architectural information can be obtained within 15 to 20 minutes after administration. Therefore, it is not necessary for the patient to return after 24 hours for scanning, as is the case when using iodide. This is of extreme importance when surgery is contemplated on the next day.

Scanning Technique. Technetium, 1 to 2 mCi., is given orally. The patient is placed on the scan table with neck extended and head immobilized. The thyroid area is scanned within 15 to 30 minutes after the dose has been administered, with the detecting probe moving toward the suprasternal notch. The time of actual sequential scanning is less than five minutes.

The gamma ray spectrometer has been peaked to accept the specific gamma energy of technetium, with the lower and upper window settings at 110 and 170 kev., respectively; a low-energy, fine-focus collimator is used. Scan speed is 100 cm. per minute; density, 75; high voltage, 1,300; and line spacing, 2 mm.

Selenomethionine

One of the amino acids, methionine, contains sulfur in its molecule. Selenium is similar to sulfur and can replace sulfur in the methionine molecule without altering the properties of the amino acid. The formula is:

$$CH_3-Se-CH_2-CH_2-CHNH_2-COOH$$

[75]Se-selenomethionine is a gamma-emitting compound and is incorporated into cells according to the rate of protein synthesis, that is, reflecting mitotic activity and cellularity.[51, 55] Selenium-75 has a physical half-life of 120 days and an effective half-life of 56 days. On disintegra-

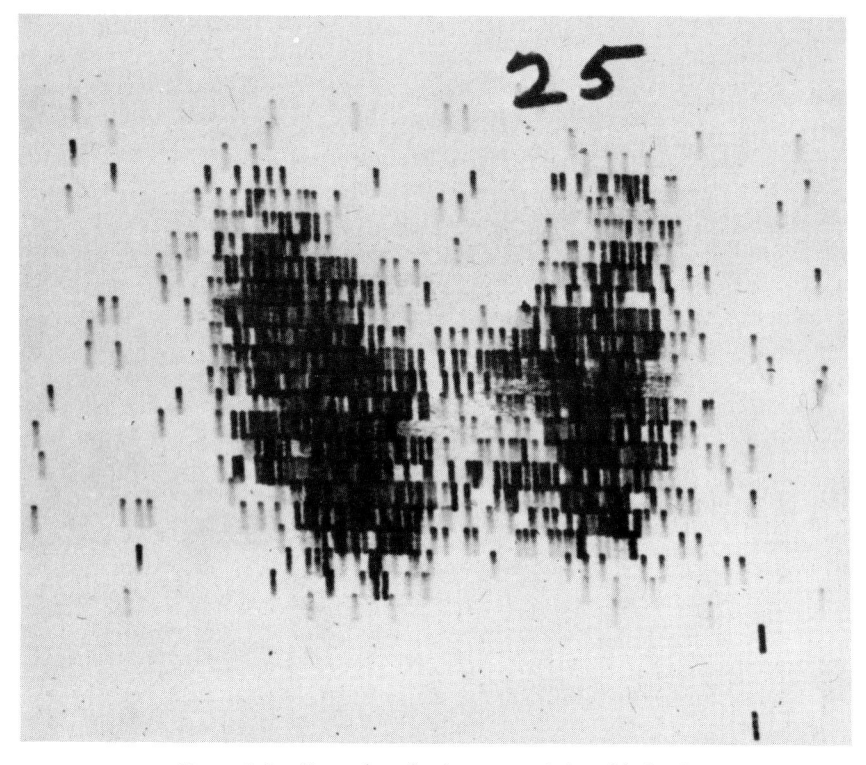

Figure 6-2. Frontal projection, normal thyroid gland.

tion, the principal gamma ray has an energy of 0.279 Mev. The average energy of the beta particle is 0.01 Mev.

The spectrometer has been peaked to accept the specific gamma energy of ^{75}Se with the lower and upper window settings at 230 and 330 kev., respectively.

The thyroid gland is initially scanned following an oral dose of 30 μCi. of [131]I. If a nonfunctioning "cool" or "cold" nodule is demonstrated, the patient next receives an intravenous dose of 150 to 250 μCi. ^{75}Se-selenomethionine. The thyroid scan is repeated 30 to 60 minutes later. The results of this technique will be discussed under the "cold" nodule.

MORPHOLOGIC CONSIDERATIONS

The Normal Thyroid

"A thyroid gland has a high probability of being normal if it has a frontal plane area less than 20 sq. cm., if all borders of both lobes are convex and if the radioactivity is uniformly distributed" (Fig. 6-2).[45]

The Abnormal Thyroid

"In a gland with a frontal area greater than 30 sq. cm., or with irregular borders or with nonuniform distribution of activity within the gland, the thyroid is probably abnormal."[45]

Extracervical Thyroid Tissue

It is of extreme importance to remember embryologic sites of thyroid tissue to avoid the labeling "metastatic disease." These areas of tissue are normally extracervical: the base of the tongue, the thyroglossal duct tract, and the retrosternal region in the elderly patient.

The lingual thyroid is a relatively rare condition and clinically presents as a moderately firm mass on the posterior aspect of the tongue. Additional thyroid tissue may or may not be palpable in the normal cervical region.

An oral dose of 20 μCi. of ^{131}I is administered; 24 hours later the patient is examined in the supine and lateral positions. Radioactivity is recorded over the posterior portion of the tongue.[19]

Thyroid Metastatic Disease

We know that the total removal of the thyroid gland will increase the avidity of metastatic foci for the radioactive iodine. Indeed, it is virtually impossible to detect metastatic lesions while thyroid tissue is still in the neck.

A tracer dose of 1,000 to 2,000 μCi. of sodium iodide-131 is administered orally 24 hours before the area of concern is to be scanned. The previous administration of thyroid-stimulating hormone (TSH) may or may not increase the uptake of ^{131}I by the metastatic tissue; this is still a controversial point.

Pulmonary Metastases. The patient is examined in the supine position with the detecting probe moving across the chest and covering an area extending from the suprasternal notch above to the costal margins in the axillary lines below. Isotopic accumulations are normally detected in the cardiac pool (left ventricle), the gastric mucosa, and the liver. Otherwise, any focus of isotopic localization within the confines of the thorax must be considered a site of metastatic disease arising from well differentiated thyroidal carcinoma.[28] This is illustrated in Case 12 (Fig. 6–13). Both ^{131}I and ^{99m}TcO$_4^-$ have been used to detect metastatic thyroid carcinoma. However, it is possible to miss metastatic thyroid tissue in the mediastinum with the use of ^{99m}TcO$_4^-$ alone. This is apparently related to the high background counting rate from the great vessels of the mediastinum. Otherwise, no difficulties have been experienced in demonstrating functioning thyroid tissue.[32] Additional investigation has shown that ^{99m}Tc may be extremely useful in that it may localize in *nonfunctional* metastatic thyroid carcinoma.[53]

Skeletal Metastases. Thyroid carcinoma is one of the several primary malignant lesions that produce osteolytic lesions in bones (other primary malignant lesions include bronchogenic, mammary, and renal carcinoma). The metastatic mass concentrates the radioiodine and presents as a "hot" focus of activity.[48] This phenomenon is described in Figures 6-14 and 6-15.

NODULATION

It is generally accepted that perhaps the chief value of thyroid imaging lies in the detection of a nodule and the establishing of a uniformity of function, that is, whether "hot" or "cold."[9, 10, 44] The requirements for detection include:[7] (1) the nodule must be large enough to produce a significant change in counting rate; (2) the nodule must result in the displacement or replacement of normally functioning tissue; and (3) the functional state of the nodule must be significantly different from the remainder of the gland.

THE "HOT" NODULE

Miller et al.[34, 35] have defined the "hot" nodule and the "cold" nodule in great detail. I shall quote them extensively: "All the following conditions would qualify as 'hot nodules' as currently defined:

(a) The autonomous hyperfunctioning thyroid lesion.

(b) Tissue of relatively normal function with surrounding areas of degeneration or thyroiditis.

(c) A normal, hyperplastic, or nodular lobe with congenital or acquired absence of the other lobe. 'Acquired' includes total or subtotal surgical resection.

(d) A prominently lobulated gland with sufficient asymmetry that by virtue of greater mass alone one lobe or one area contains significantly more radioactive iodine than the other. (Toxic dependent goiter [Graves' disease] may present in such a fashion.)"[34, 35]

"Hot" nodules are considered benign. However, from time to time investigators have described a carcinoma occurring in a gland containing a "hot" nodule. The lateral cervical scan is of utmost importance in defining the anteroposterior dimension of the thyroid gland. It is possible that the focus of increased activity, represented by a "hot" nodule, lying spatially anterior or posterior to the area of malignant degeneration (which malignancy itself presents as a "cold" nodule), will obscure the "cold" nodule. An incidental carcinoma has been reported in a "hot" nodule by Becker et al.[11] and by Meadows.[31] Apparently such neoplasms have been reported as occurring in the same gland with "hot" nodules.[37] Shimaoka and Sokal[49] have written about the differentiation of benign and malignant nodules. Dische[18] described a carcinoma in which the malignant tumor was the hyperfunctioning tissue. However, the general conclusion is that while thyroid carcinoma may be associated with a solitary hyperfunctioning nodule, this is very infrequent.

That function is autonomous may be shown by one or both of two methods:

1. If function is present in extranodular tissue, that is, function is not localized to the nodule, administer 0.3 mg. of thyroxine daily for 14 days. A repeat scan will demonstrate suppression, complete or partial, of the extranodular function.

2. If function is virtually localized to the nodule, that is, there is no extranodular function, administer 10 units of TSH. A repeat scan will demonstrate function in the formerly suppressed tissue equal to that of the nodule, that is, there has been selective stimulation by TSH of suppressed normal tissue.[34]

Miller and Block[33] have again defined the problem of the "hot" nodule as follows: "First the functioning nodule itself, as defined below, has correlated to date with a benign histologic pattern,[34] and second, secretory activity may or may not produce a hyperthyroid state."[36]

McCormack and Sheline[30] use the term hyperfunction as follows: "On a gram for gram basis, the tissue of concern appeared to be functioning at a rate in excess of that in the extranodular tissue. It implies nothing with respect to the clinical state of the patient."

The "Cool" and "Cold" Nodules

If a circumscribed area shows less activity than the surrounding tissue, that is, it is a partially functioning nodule, it is considered a "cool" nodule. If the area shows no activity, it is termed a "cold" nodule.

Again, I refer to the excellent investigation of Miller and associates[35] and, in general, will use their classification.

Class 1. In the nondelineated nodule, the thyroid scan appears normal, and localization marks alone serve to identify the position of the nodule.

Class 2. The nodule delineated by size alone appears as an enlarged area, but the average density of the radioactivity equals that of the normal lobe.

Class 3. The nodule is delineated by means of location adjacent to the lobe, that is, the nodule replaces a portion of the lobe.

Class 4. The nodule is demarcated as an area of diminished function within the outline of the thyroid.

Histologically the area of diminished-to-absent radioactivity may represent an adenoma, cyst, hematoma, localized thyroiditis, congenital absence of part of the thyroid,[20] or carcinoma[31, 37] or lymphoma.[50]

Harrison[24] described his experience with a series of 1,200 patients undergoing thyroidectomy at the Medical College of Virginia Hospitals. He noted that of 288 patients with a single "cold" nodule, 31 had a malignant condition, for a malignancy rate of 11 percent, and of 55 patients with multiple "cold" nodules, 10 had a malignant condition, for a malignancy rate of 18 percent. He concluded that 12 percent of "cold" nodules were malignant.

Harrison[24] has further summarized his findings: (1) The thyroid scan is valuable and should be performed before thyroid surgery. (2) Carcinoma occurs primarily in the "cold" nodule; therefore, the "cold" nodule should be removed. (3) The "hot" nodule should be removed if there has been no response to thyroid extract. (4) Therefore, it is of utmost importance to determine whether or not the nodule or nodules are "hot" or "cold" on the scan. (5) The lateral cervical scan is important for correct interpretation.

It is generally accepted that large numbers of those nodules removed because of the possibility of malignant degeneration are benign. A technique[55] has been developed whereby a thyroid scan using ^{75}Se-selenomethionine was performed after a standard ^{131}I scan had revealed a "cold" nodule. These two scans were complementary in that if the "cold" nodule by ^{131}I were "hot" with ^{75}Se-selenomethionine, there was one chance out of two that this nodule was malignant. However, the authors showed that thyroiditis will also increase the uptake of ^{75}Se-selenomethionine. Nevertheless, this technique will undoubtedly lead to a more accurate preoperative tissue diagnosis of the "cold" nodule.

ASSOCIATED ENDOCRINOPATHIES

Hyperparathyroidism

It has been shown that surgical lesions of the parathyroid and thyroid glands may coexist; therefore, the patient undergoing a surgical procedure for either should be evaluated before and during the operation for abnormalities in the other gland.[26]

Pheochromocytoma

Although the association of medullary carcinoma of the thyroid and pheochromocytoma is uncommon, nevertheless, a patient with one of these conditions should be examined for the other.[13, 14]

PHYSIOLOGICAL CONSIDERATIONS

Assessment of Thyroid Function

It is beyond the scope of this chapter to discuss in detail (1) the direct tests of thyroid function, (2) tests of hormones in the blood and (3) peripheral hormone action. These studies have been described by

Hamolsky and associates,[21, 22] Sisson,[52] Selenkow and Refetoff,[47] Ashkar and Smith,[6] Werner and Ingbar,[58] Heck and Gottschalk,[25] and Atkins and Richards.[8]

Briefly, the iodide ion is trapped by the thyroid gland and then, along with the amino acid, tyrosine, undergoes conversion to the hormones triiodothyronine (T3) and thyroxine (T4). These hormones are subsequently released into the circulation to exert their metabolic effects on the peripheral tissues.

Normal extrathyroidal sites of iodine concentration in the body within the first 24 hours include the salivary glands and saliva, the stomach, the urine (urinary bladder), and the colon.

Thyroid Uptake Study. The radioactive iodine (most commonly ^{131}I) is administered orally. Usually 24 hours later (less commonly at 6 or 12 hours), the activity in the neck region is measured as a percentage of the administered dose. Radioactive iodine remains the agent of choice for determining thyroidal uptake.[56]

Example: The patient swallows a 20-μCi. capsule of sodium radioiodide (^{131}I). A capsule from the same shipment is selected as a standard. The standard and the administered dose decay at presumably the same rate. However, it has been known that variations in the capsule content of the tracer dose do occur on occasion. Therefore, each lot of capsules should be precounted.[27] Hence, we have only to compare the counts per unit of time from the standard capsule with those from the patient's thyroid gland under similar conditions of geometry to arrive at a percentage of the ingested dose taken up by the gland.

Laboratory Background
Two readings   231 counts per 2 min.

$$\frac{+265}{496}$$

Average = 248 counts per 2 min.

Standard Capsule at 30 cm. from Detecting Probe

Two readings   7,868 counts per 2 min.

$$\frac{+8,037}{15,905}$$

Average = 7,952 counts per 2 min.

Patient's Neck at 30 cm. from Detecting Probe

Two readings   2,558 counts per 2 min.

$$\frac{+2,514}{5,072}$$

Average = 2,536 counts per 2 min.

Calculations:

$$\frac{\text{Standard}}{\text{Background}} = \frac{7{,}952}{-248}$$
$$\overline{7{,}704} \text{ counts per 2 min., representing 100 percent}$$

$$\frac{\text{Patient}}{\textit{Background}} = \frac{2{,}536}{-248}$$
$$\overline{2{,}288} \text{ counts per 2 min.}$$

$$\frac{7{,}704}{100} = \frac{2{,}288}{X} \quad X = 29.7 \text{ per cent}$$

INTERPRETATION. It is generally accepted that thyroid activity corresponding to less than 15 percent of the dose reflects hypothyroidism, and an activity of more than 45 percent is an indication of hyperthyroidism.

Hamolsky[21] has listed factors that either increase or decrease iodide uptake. The factors *increasing* uptake are acute renal failure and low dietary intake of iodine. Those factors *decreasing* iodide uptake are dietary (turnips, rhubarb), chemicals (thiocyanate, chlorate, periodate, iodate, nitrate, and perchlorate), and drugs (thiourea, desiccated thyroid, thyroxine, and possibly corticosteroids).

Thyroid Suppression Test. A 24-hour radioactive iodine uptake study is performed. The patient then receives triiodothyronine four times daily for seven days. The 24-hour radioactive iodine uptake study is then repeated.

INTERPRETATION. Normally the second radioactive iodine uptake will be depressed. In the borderline case of hyperthyroidism, however, the second uptake study will not be depressed.

Primary Versus Secondary Myxedema. This study allows us to differentiate primary thyroid deficiency from secondary thyroid deficiency seen in hypopituitarism. A 24-hour radioactive iodine uptake is performed.

INTERPRETATION. The 24-hour uptake is reduced, reflecting nonspecific hypothyroidism. The patient then receives TSH (10 units intramuscularly daily for three days), and the 24-hour uptake study is repeated.

The second 24-hour uptake remains low, despite the administration of TSH, if the thyroid gland itself is at fault. This, therefore, represents primary thyroid deficiency. If the uptake is increased after the administration of TSH, the thyroid gland itself is normal and the pituitary gland is at fault.

Conversion Ratio. The conversion ratio is the percentage of circulating radioactivity already in hormonal form. The following is the protocol outlined by Hamolsky:[21] The plasma protein precipitable ^{131}I divided by the total plasma ^{131}I times 100 is determined 24 hours after the administration of a tracer dose of iodine. This ratio varies from 13 to 42 percent in the euthyroid state and is above 45 percent in the hyperthyroid state.

Triiodothyronine (T3) (Thyrobinding Index). This is the "Hamolsky test" and depends on the fact that free T3 will bind to red blood cells, clay, and ion-exchange resins. It is an indirect measure of thyroid activity since it measures the relative percentage of unsaturation of the patient's thyroxine-binding globulin (TBG).

Commercially available radioactive T3 is added to a small volume (usually several milliliters) of patient's blood and incubated. The proportion of radioactive T3 that remains bound to the red blood cells is then determined. Normally the red blood cell uptake is between 11 and 17 percent. In hyperthyroidism, more thyroid hormone is available for binding by red blood cells or resins. Therefore, the red blood cell uptake is greater than 17 percent. In contrast, the red blood cell uptake is lower in the hypothyroid state. This is because of a greater binding avidity of T3 to plasma proteins. Therefore, a lesser amount of T3 is available for binding by the red blood cells.

Some conditions that may spuriously *increase* T3 uptake have been described;[21] they include nephrosis, severe liver disease, metastatic malignant disease, anticoagulation, and metabolic and respiratory acidosis. Conditions that *decrease* T3 uptake are found in patients with hyperthyroidism receiving iodide or propylthiouracil, those being given estrogen, and those who are pregnant, beginning toward the latter part of the first trimester.

T4 Test. Since a single test such as the standard T3 procedure does not necessarily give all the information required, the concomitant use of the T4 test has been developed.

The Murphy-Pattee T4[38-40] study offers a direct measurement of thyroid function by determining the total serum thyroxin: that which is bound to the thyroxine-binding proteins plus the free circulating thyroxine. Hence, this study provides a *direct* measure of the output of the thyroid gland.

INTERPRETATION. Murphy and Pattee[40] have reported values for thyroxine uncorrected for extraction efficiency. It is necessary to divide by their extraction efficiency factor of 0.77 to convert their values to corrected values.

The uncorrected normal range of 4.0 to 11.0 μg. per 100 ml. is converted to the corrected normal range of 5.2 to 14.3 μg. per 100 ml. (i.e., $\frac{4.0}{0.77} = 5.2$ and $\frac{11.0}{0.77} = 14.3$). They obtained a correlation with the clinical diagnosis of 97 percent.

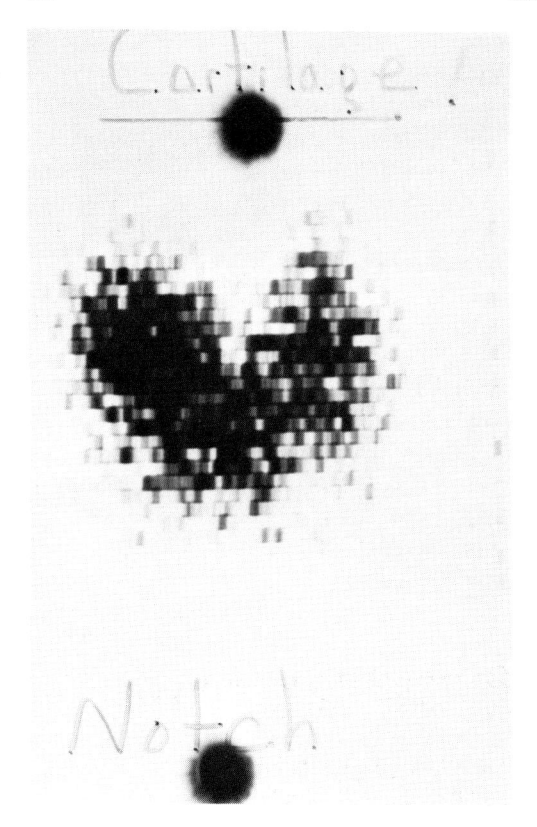

Figure 6-3. Frontal projection, multinodular goiter.

When both test values are decreased, the patient is usually hypothyroid; when both test values are increased, the patient is usually hyperthyroid; and when both test values are normal, the patient is usually euthyroid.

ILLUSTRATIVE CASES WITH DESCRIPTION OF SCANS

Case 1. A 31-year-old woman was admitted for evaluation of fatigue. The frontal photoscan (Fig. 6-2) showed the size, shape, and uniformity of isotopic localization of the normal thyroid gland.

Case 2. A 46-year-old woman with multinodular goiter was seen for follow-up study. A 2-cm. nodule was palpated in the right lobe, as was another nodule in the lower pole of the left lobe.

The frontal photoscan (Fig. 6-3) showed an area of slightly increased isotopic localization in the right lobe and an area of slightly diminished uptake in the lower portion of the left lobe, corresponding to the clinically palpable nodules. This irregular pattern of radioactivity reflects multiple nodules.

Case 3. A 66-year-old woman entered with a known substernal

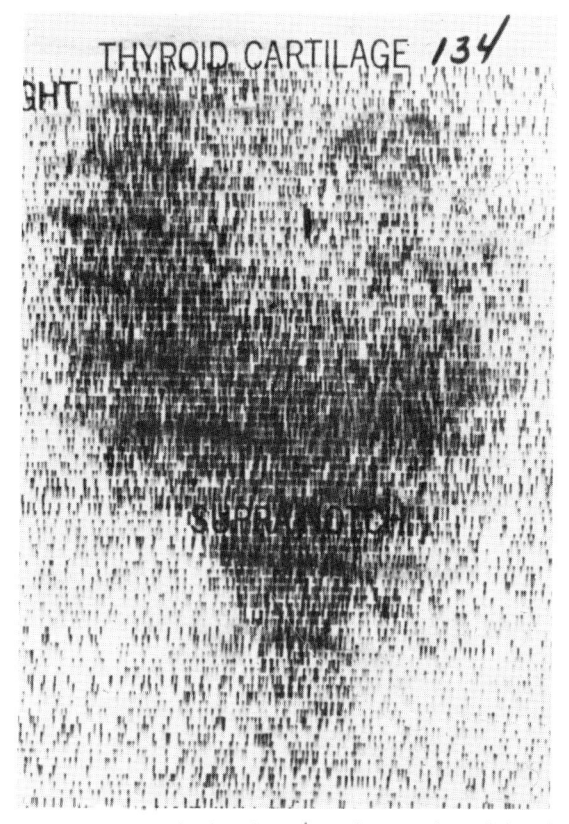

Figure 6-4. Frontal projection, intrathoracic extension of thyroid tissue.

goiter of 16 years' duration. The frontal photoscan (Fig. 6-4) showed a huge thyroid gland with diminished uptake in the region of the left lobe. Extension of thyroid tissue below the suprasternal notch has been demonstrated.

Case 4. A 52-year-old woman had had a left thyroid lobectomy some years earlier. A routine chest roentgenogram disclosed a superior mediastinal mass. The frontal photoscan (Fig. 6-5) showed a functioning right lobe of the thyroid gland and a surgically absent left lobe. A large mass of thyroid tissue inferior to the suprasternal notch has been demonstrated, representing the intrathoracic extension and corresponding to the mediastinal mass noted on the chest film.

Case 5. A 31-year-old man entered for evaluation of a mass in the inferolateral aspect of the left lobe of the thyroid. The frontal photoscan (Fig. 6-6) showed a 2-cm. area of diminished isotopic localization in the region of the clinically palpable nodule, representing a "cool" nodule. A left subtotal thyroidectomy was performed and revealed a follicular adenoma.

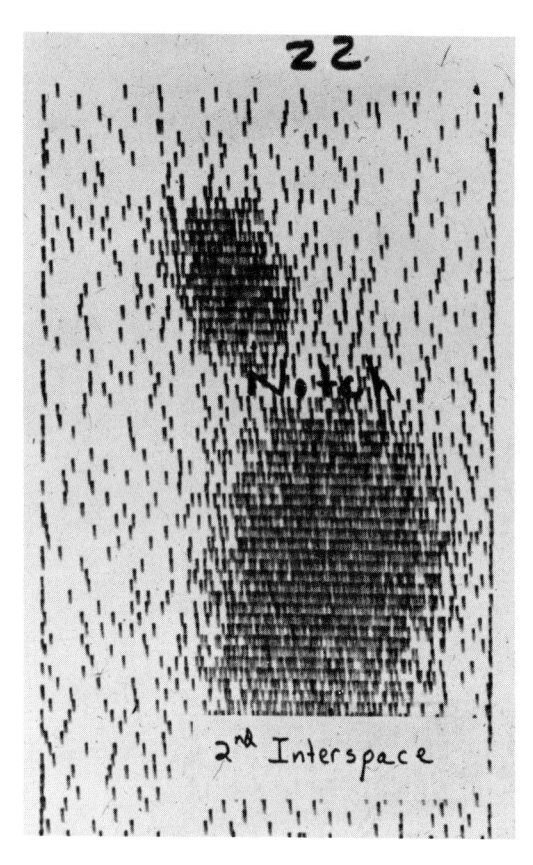

Figure 6-5. Frontal projection, functioning right lobe; surgically absent left lobe; intrathoracic extension of thyroid tissue.

Case 6. A 45-year-old woman entered for evaluation of a large (3 cm.) nodule in the left lobe of the thyroid, noted three months before admission. A frontal scan (Fig. 6-7) revealed a normal-appearing right lobe. A large area of absent activity is noted in the region of the left lobe, corresponding to the palpable nodule. A left subtotal thyroidectomy was performed and revealed a follicular adenoma.

Case 7. This 60-year-old man had had a left total thyroidectomy and radical neck dissection for papillary adenocarcinoma 12 years earlier. The frontal scan (Fig. 6-8) revealed right lobar tissue. The left lobe is surgically absent.

Case 8. This 39-year-old woman had had a left total thyroidectomy and right subtotal thyroidectomy for papillary and follicular adenocarcinoma eight months earlier. The frontal photoscan (Fig. 6-9) showed a small remnant of the right lobe. The left lobe is surgically absent.

Case 9. A 23-year-old woman entered for evaluation of a nodule in the right lobe of the thyroid gland. The frontal photoscan (Fig. 6-10) showed an irregular area of diminished-to-absent uptake in the right lobe corresponding to the clinically palpable nodule. A right subtotal

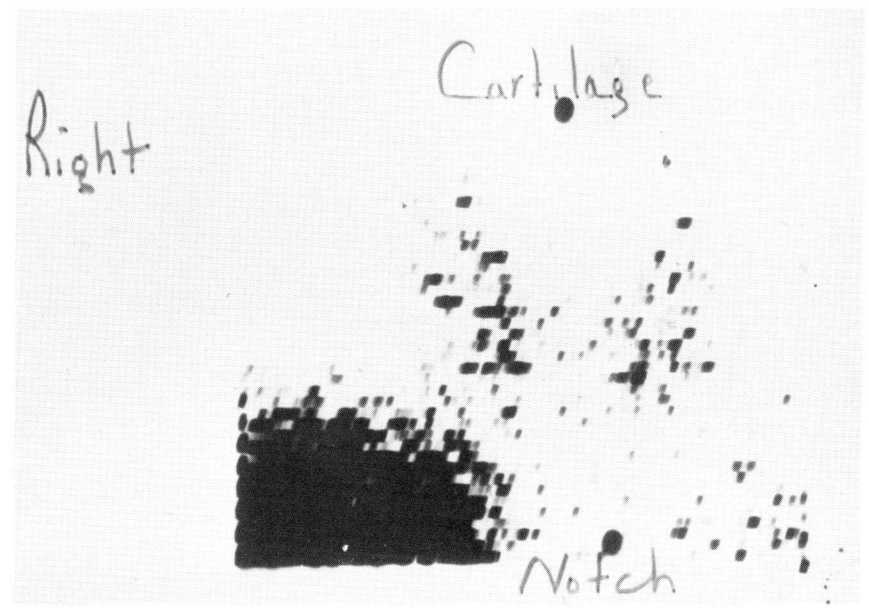

Figure 6-6. Frontal projection, 2-cm. area of diminished isotopic localization along the lower lateral border of the left lobe representing a follicular adenoma.

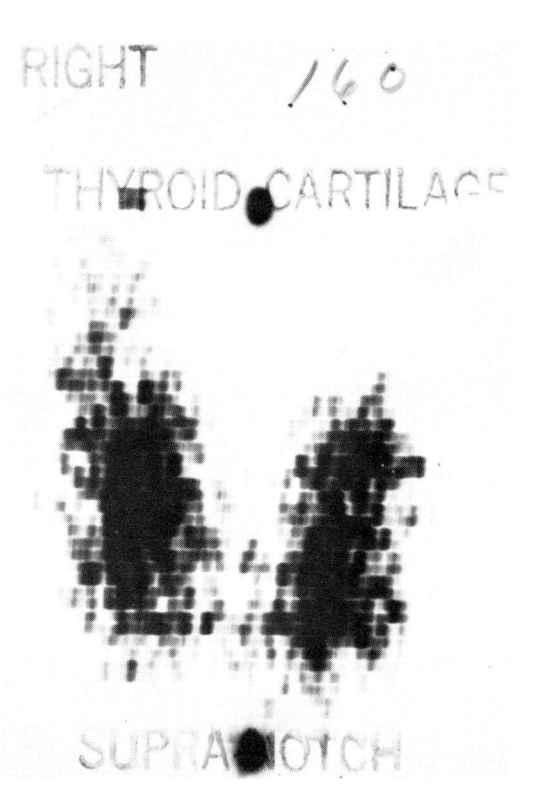

Figure 6-7. Frontal projection, a "cold" nodule, left lobe of the thyroid representing a follicular adenoma.

88　Surgery of the Thyroid Gland

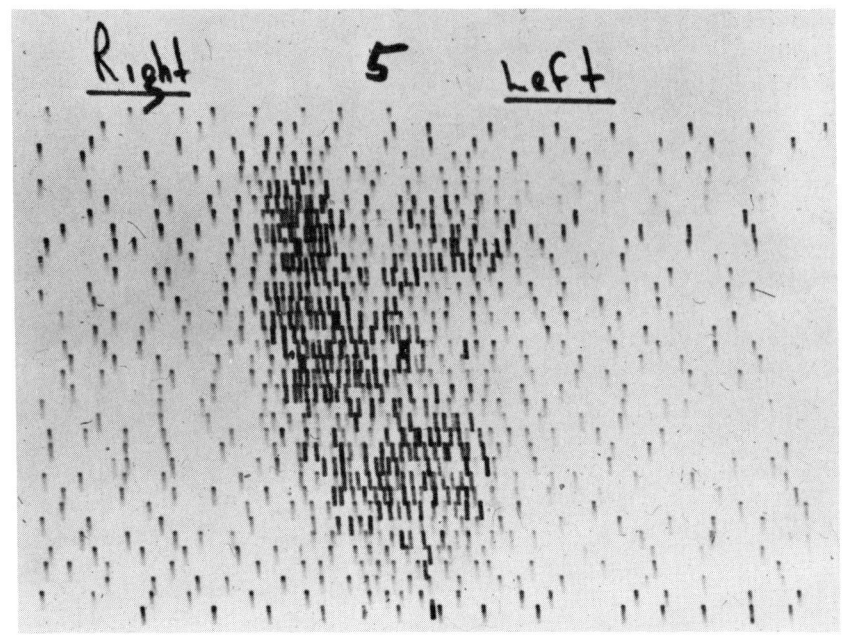

Figure 6–8.　Frontal projection, surgically absent left lobe; remnant of right lobe.

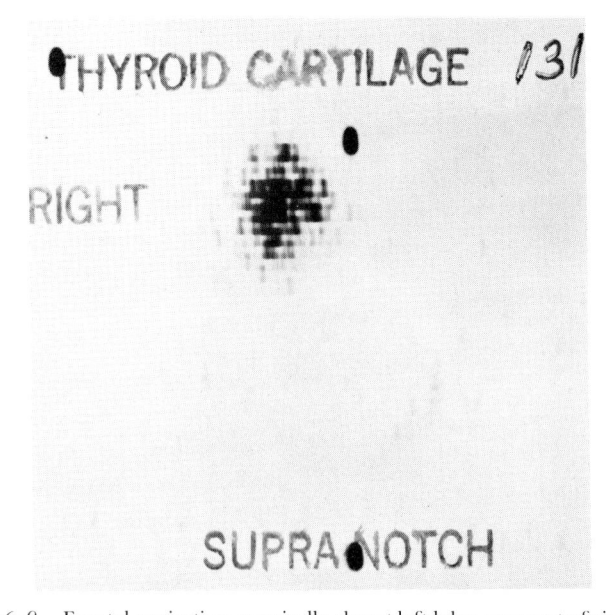

Figure 6–9.　Frontal projection, surgically absent left lobe; remnant of right lobe.

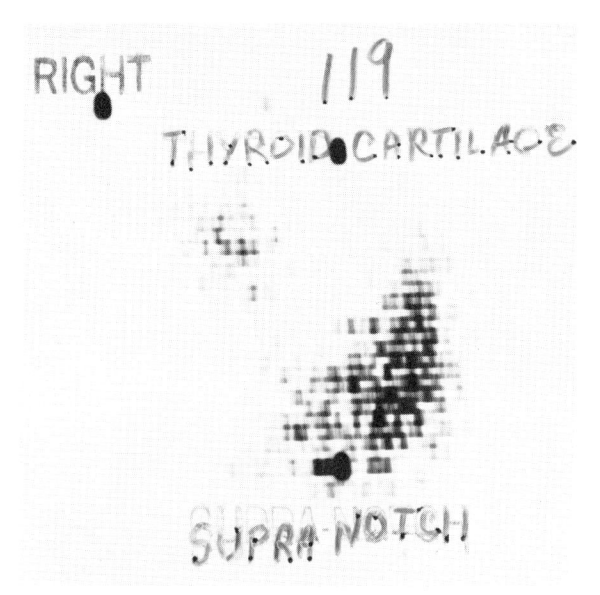

THE SURGICAL SIGNIFICANCE OF THYROID ISOTOPOLOGY 89

Figure 6–10. Frontal projection, a "cool" adenomatous nodule occupying much of the right lobe of the thyroid.

thyroidectomy was performed and revealed a benign adenomatous nodule.

Case 10. A 60-year-old woman entered for evaluation of an anterior cervical mass. The frontal scan (Fig. 6–11) revealed an enlarged thyroid gland with irregular areas of isotopic localization, representing multinodular goiter.

Case 11. This 40-year-old woman entered for evaluation of a "goiter" noted three weeks earlier. On examination, the thyroid gland was enlarged, firm, and tender. The clinical impression was acute thyroiditis.

The frontal scan (Fig. 6–12*A*) did not demonstrate radioactivity. This was consistent with the diagnosis of acute thyroiditis. The patient was given prednisone and rapidly improved clinically. A repeat thyroid scan (Fig. 6–12*B*) demonstrated a normal pattern of radioactivity.

Case 12. This 44-year-old woman had had a right total lobectomy and left subtotal thyroidectomy for a papillary carcinoma 22 years ago. Twenty-one years ago, a right radical neck dissection was performed for metastatic adenocarcinoma to the right cervical lymph nodes.

A posteroanterior chest film made during the present admission revealed extensive metastatic disease. A frontal chest scan (Fig. 6–13) revealed multiple small foci of isotopic localization throughout, especially in the lower lungs. These foci correspond to the multiple nodulations noted on the chest film and represent foci of pulmonary metastatic disease.

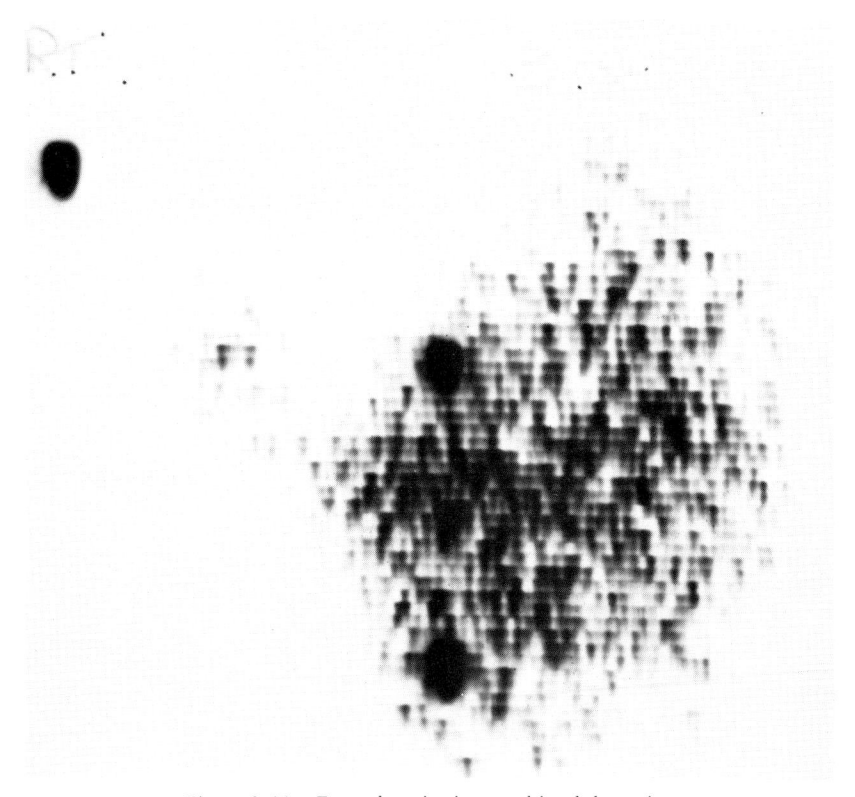

Figure 6-11. Frontal projection, multinodular goiter.

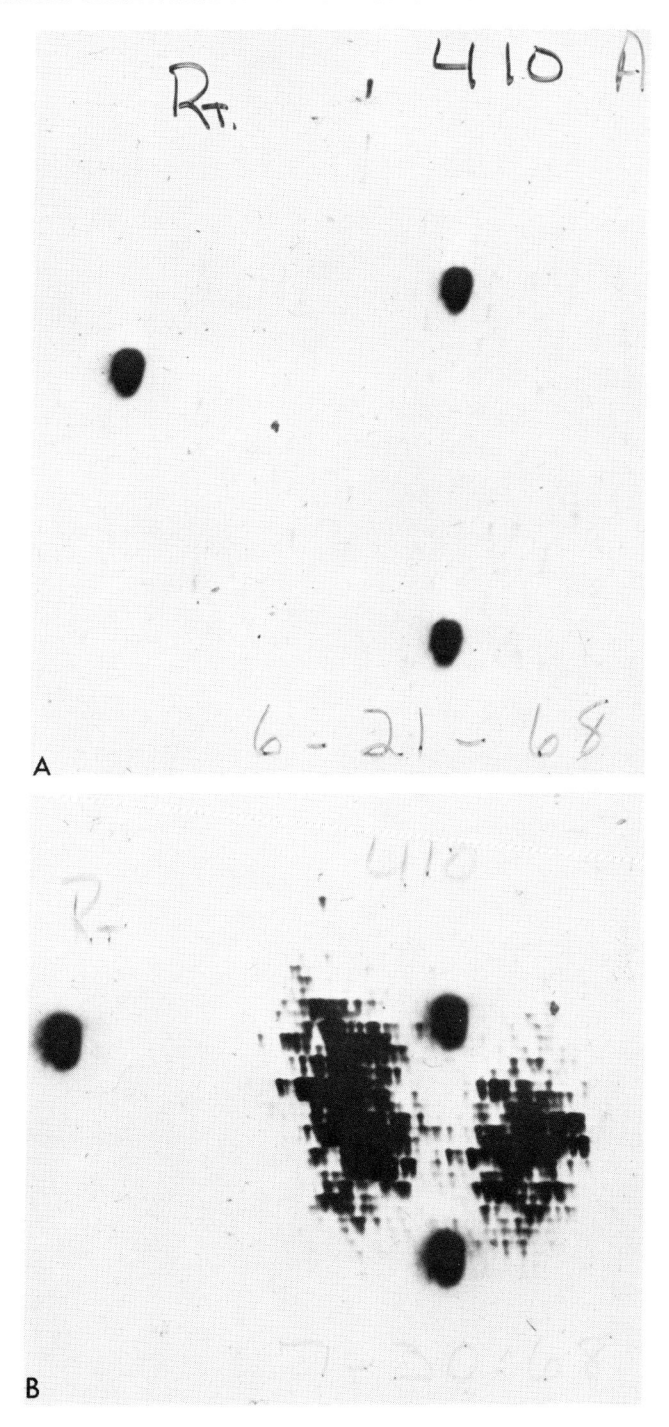

The Surgical Significance of Thyroid Isotopology

Figure 6–12. *A*, Frontal projection, no isotopic localization by thyroid tissue has been demonstrated. *B*, Frontal projection, showing satisfactory pattern of radioactivity following treatment with prednisone.

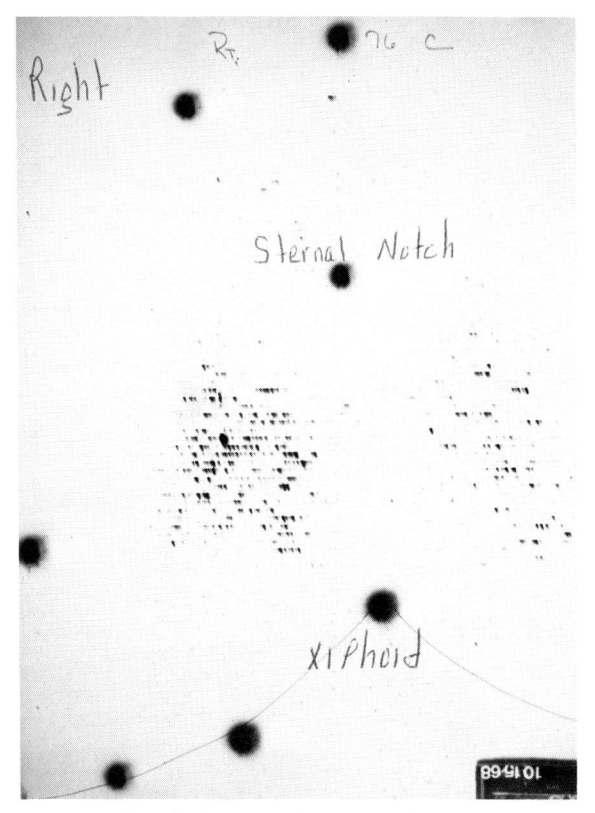

Figure 6-13. Frontal projection, thyroid area; foci of functioning thyroid tissue to the right of the midline. Chest, multiple small foci of isotopic localization, especially at the bases, representing nodulations of metastatic disease to the lung.

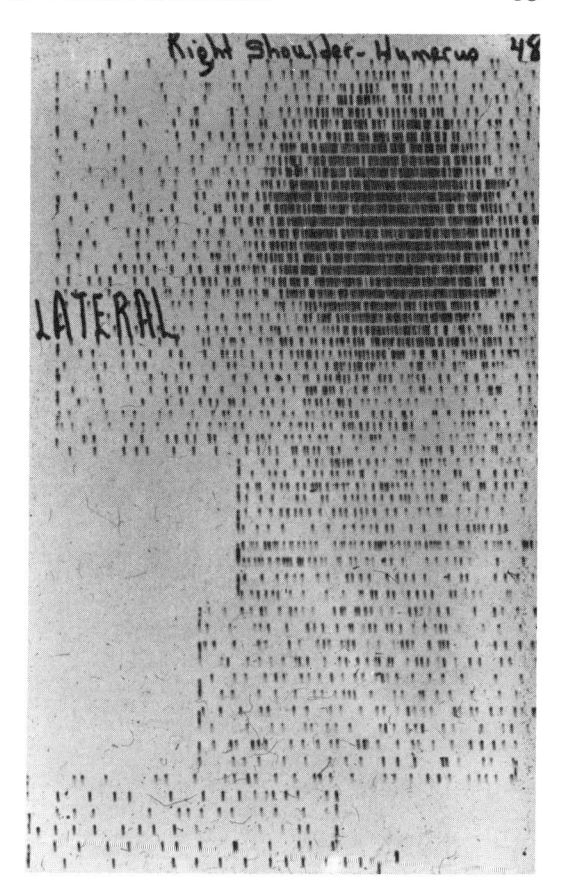

THE SURGICAL SIGNIFICANCE OF THYROID ISOTOPOLOGY 93

Figure 6-14. Frontal projection, upper right humerus showing isotopic localization by focus of metastatic tissue from the thyroid.

Case 13. This 71-year-old man had had a total thyroidectomy for adenocarcinoma. A metastatic series demonstrated destructive changes involving the upper right humeral shaft and the right acetabular region.

A cervical scan failed to demonstrate any thyroid tissue. The frontal photoscan of the right humerus (Fig. 6-14) showed a focus of isotopic localization corresponding to the osteolytic lesion and representing a nidus of metastatic disease from he thyroid. The frontal photoscan of the right hemipelvis (Fig. 6-15) demonstrated isotopic localization in the right acetabular region, corresponding to the destructive metastatic lesion.

Case 14. This 62-year-old woman was admitted for thyroidectomy for toxic goiter after three months of therapy with propylthiouracil. Posteroanterior and lateral films of the chest showed no evidence of lung disease. The trachea was deviated to the right, secondary to enlargement of the left lobe of the thyroid gland. The frontal scan (Fig. 6-16) revealed an enlarged left lobe of the thyroid. No activity was demonstrated in the region of the right lobe.

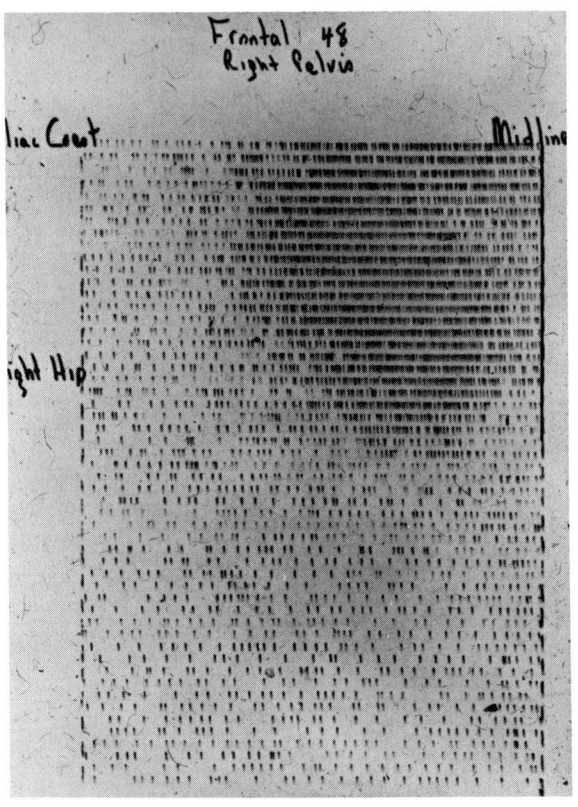

Figure 6-15. Frontal projection, right hemipelvis, demonstrating isotopic localization by metastatic thyroid tissue.

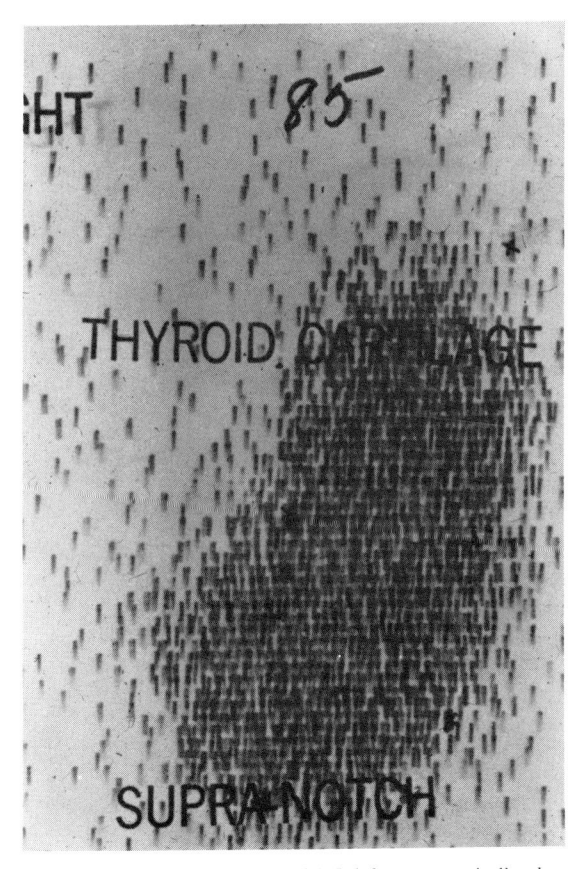

Figure 6-16. Frontal projection, enlarged left lobe; congenitally absent right lobe.

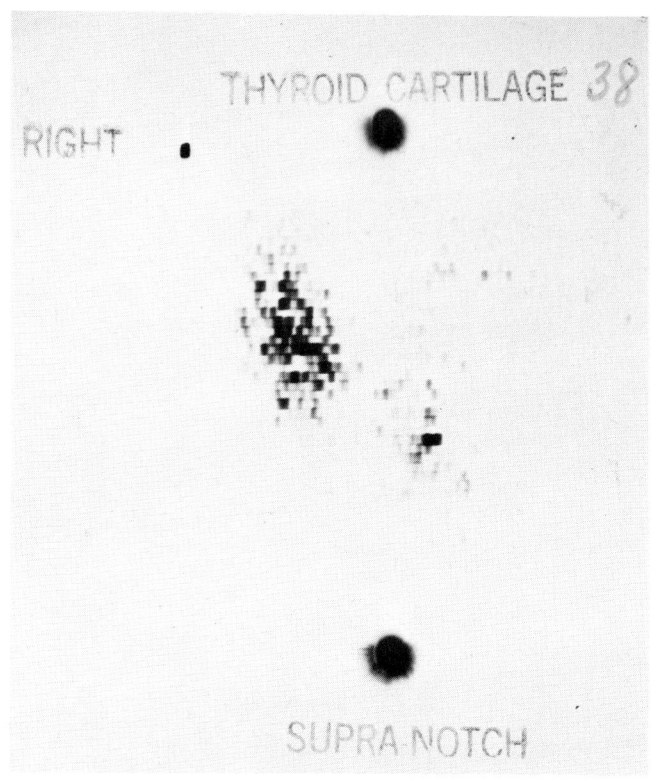

Figure 6–17. Frontal projection, almost total absence of activity, left lobe of thyroid, representing partially cystic follicular adenoma.

At the time of surgery the left thyroid lobe and isthmus were enlarged about three times normal and were nodular. Sections revealed adenomatous goiter with secondary hyperplasia. The right lobe of the thyroid gland was completely absent. There was no evidence of any remnant or underdevelopment of the right thyroid lobe. This was considered a congenital absence of the right thyroid lobe.

Case 15. This 44-year-old woman entered for evaluation of a nodule in the left lobe of the thyroid. A frontal scan (Fig. 6–17) demonstrated almost total absence of activity in the region of the left lobe. A left total thyroidectomy was performed and revealed a partially cystic (5 × 6 cm.) follicular adenoma, Hürthle cell type.

REFERENCES

1. Andros, G., Harper, P. V., Lathrop, K. A., et al.: Pertechnetate-99m localization in man with applications to thyroid scanning and the study of thyroid physiology. J. Clin. Endocr. 25:1067–1076 (Aug.) 1965.
2. Anger, H. O.: Gamma ray and positron scintillation camera. Nucleonics 21:56–59 (Oct.) 1963.
3. Anger, H. O.: Sensitivity, resolution, and linearity of the scintillation camera. A.E.C.

No. UCRL-16724, University of California, Lawrence Radiation Laboratory, February, 1966.
4. Anger, H. O.: Radioisotope cameras. In Hine, G. J. (ed.): Instrumentation in Nuclear Medicine. New York, Academic Press, Inc., 1967, pp. 485–552.
5. Anger, H. O., and Davis, D. H.: Gamma ray detection efficiency and image resolution in sodium iodide. Rev. Sci. Inst. 35:693–697 (June) 1964.
6. Ashkar, F. S., and Smith, E. M.: The dynamic thyroid study. A rapid evaluation of thyroid functioning and anatomy using ^{99m}Tc as pertechnetate. J.A.M.A. 217:441–446 (July 26) 1971.
7. Atkins, H. L., and Fleay, R. F.: Data blending with ^{99m}Tc in evaluating thyroid anatomy by scintillation scanning. J. Nucl. Med. 9:66–73 (Feb.) 1968.
8. Atkins, H. L., and Richards, P.: Assessment of thyroid function and anatomy with technetium-99m as pertechnetate. J. Nucl. Med. 9:7–15 (Jan.) 1968.
9. Attie, J. N.: The use of radioactive iodine in the evaluation of thyroid nodules. Surgery 47:611–614 (April) 1960.
10. Bartels, E. C., Bell, G. O., and Geokas, M. C.: Evaluation of the thyroid nodule. S. Clin. N. Amer. 42:655–665 (June) 1962.
11. Becker, F. O., Economou, P. G., and Schwartz, T. B.: The occurrence of carcinoma in "hot" thyroid nodules: Report of two cases. Ann. Intern. Med. 58:877–882 (May) 1963.
12. Best, E. B., and McKenney, J. F.: Thyroid scanning: Clinical approach. Postgrad. Med. 39: A 87–96 (May) 1966.
13. Block, M. A.: Medullary thyroid carcinoma: A component of an interesting endocrine syndrome. CA 19:74–79 (March-April) 1969.
14. Block, M. A., Miller, J. M., and Horn, R. C., Jr.: Medullary carcinoma of the thyroid: Surgical implications. Arch. Surg. 96:521–526 (April) 1968.
15. Cassen, B., Curtis, L., Reed, R., et al.: Instrumentation for I^{131} use in medical studies. Nucleonics 9:46–50 (Aug.) 1951.
16. Charkes, N. D., and Sklaroff, D. M.: The use of iodine 125 in thyroid scintiscanning. Amer. J. Roentgen. 90:1052–1058 (Nov.) 1963.
17. Collica, C. J., Robinson, T., and Hayt, D. B.: Comparative study of the gamma camera and rectilinear scanner. Amer. J. Roentgen. 100:761–779 (Aug.) 1967.
18. Dische, S.: The radioisotope scan applied to the detection of carcinoma in thyroid swellings. Cancer 17:473–479 (April) 1964.
19. Dodds, W. J., and Powell, M. R.: Lingual thyroid scanned with technetium 99m pertechnetate: Report of two cases. Amer. J. Roentgen. 100:786–791 (Aug.) 1967.
20. Hamburger, J. I., and Hamburger, S. W.: Thyroidal hemiagenesis: Report of a case and comments on clinical ramifications. Arch. Surg. 100:319–320 (March) 1970.
21. Hamolsky, M. W.: Radioisotopic tests of thyroid function. Lahey Clin. Found. Bull. 16:313–319, 1967.
22. Hamolsky, M. W., Koplowitz, J. M., and Solomon, D. H.: Measurement of thyroid function. In Blahd, W. H. (ed.): Nuclear Medicine. New York, The Blakiston Division, McGraw-Hill Book Company, 1965, pp. 185–258.
23. Harper, P. V., Lathrop, K. A., Jiminez, F., et al.: Technetium 99m as a scanning agent. Radiology 85:101–109 (July) 1965.
24. Harrison, J. M.: Presented at the Postgraduate Course "Nuclear Medicine" sponsored by Department of Radiology, Medical College of Virginia, Feb. 27–March 2, 1968.
25. Heck, L. L., and Gottschalk, A.: A rapid and reproducible method for ^{99m}Tc thyroid uptake. J. Nucl. Med. 11:325 (June) 1970.
26. Laing, V. O., Fram, B., and Block, M. A.: Associated primary hyperparathyroidism and thyroid lesions. Surgical considerations. Arch. Surg. 98:709–712 (June) 1969.
27. Lawrence, C. A., Russel, M. E., Davis, R. P., et al.: The effect of capsule content variations on thyroid uptake results. J. Nucl. Med. 11:561–563 (Sept.) 1970.
28. Llewellyn, T., Jansen, C., Ridings, G. R., et al.: Roentgenographically undetectable pulmonary metastases from thyroid carcinoma demonstrated by lung scan. Radiology 91:753–754 (Oct.) 1968.
29. McAllister, J. D., Alexander, G. H., Goldberg, H. E., et al.: The clinical application of the Anger gamma camera to diseases of the thyroid. Amer. J. Roentgen. 100:780–785 (Aug.) 1967.
30. McCormack, K. R., and Sheline, G. E.: Long-term studies of solitary autonomous thyroid nodules. J. Nucl. Med. 8:701–708 (Oct.) 1967.
31. Meadows, P. M.: Scintillation scanning in the management of the clinically single thyroid nodule. J.A.M.A. 177:229–234 (July 29) 1961.

32. Meighan, J. W., and Dworkin, H. J.: Failure to detect ^{131}I positive thyroid metastases with [99m]Tc. J. Nucl. Med. 11:173–174 (April) 1970.
33. Miller, J. M., and Block, M. A.: The autonomous functioning thyroid nodule. Therapeutic considerations. Arch. Surg. 96:386–393 (March) 1968.
34. Miller, J. M., and Hamburger, J. I.: The thyroid scintigram. I. The hot nodule. Radiology 84:66–73 (Jan.) 1965.
35. Miller, J. M., Hamburger, J. I., and Mellinger, R. C.: The thyroid scintigram. II. The cold nodule. Radiology 85:702–710 (Oct.) 1965.
36. Miller, J. M., Horn, R. C., and Block, M. A.: The evolution of toxic nodular goiter. Arch. Intern. Med. 113:72–88 (Jan.) 1964.
37. Molnar, G. D., Childs, D. S., Jr., and Woolner, L. B.: Histologic evidence of malignancy in a thyroid gland bearing a hot nodule. J. Clin. Endocr. 18:1132–1134 (Oct.) 1958.
38. Murphy, B. E.: The determination of thyroxine by competitive protein-binding analysis employing an ion-exchange resin and radiothyroxine. J. Lab. Clin. Med. 66:161–167 (July) 1965.
39. Murphy, B. E., and Pattee, C. J.: Determination of thyroxine utilizing the property of protein-binding. J. Clin. Endocr. 24:187–196 (Feb.) 1964.
40. Murphy, B. E., Pattee, C. J., and Gold, A.: Clinical evaluation of a new method for the determination of serum thyroxine. J. Clin. Endocr. 26:247–256 (March) 1966.
41. Murray, P., and Thomson, J. A.: The use of the gamma camera in the investigation of thyroid disorders. Amer. J. Roentgen. 90:345–351 (Aug.) 1963.
42. Norcross, J. W., and Siber, F. J.: Thyroid scanography. Lahey Clin. Found. Bull. 17:63–66 (Jan.-March) 1968.
43. Quinn, J. L., 3rd, and Behinfar, M.: Radioisotope scanning of the thyroid. J.A.M.A. 199:920–924 (March 20) 1967.
44. Rawson, R. W., Skanse, B. N., Marinelli, L. D., et al.: Radioactive iodine; its use in studying certain functions of normal and neoplastic thyroid tissues. Cancer 2:279–292 (March) 1949.
45. Renda, F., Holmes, R. A., North, W. A., et al.: Characteristics of thyroid scans in normal persons, hyperthyroidism and nodular goiter. J. Nucl. Med. 9:156–159 (April) 1968.
46. Sanders, T. P., and Kuhl, D. E.: Technetium pertechnetate as a thyroid scanning agent. Radiology 91:23–26 (July) 1968.
47. Selenkow, H. A., and Refetoff, S.: Common tests of thyroid function in serum. J.A.M.A. 202:153–154 (Oct. 9) 1967.
48. Shahani, S. N., Sharma, S. M., Ganatra, R. D., et al.: Functioning metastasis from thyroid cancer. Arch. Surg. 95:689–692 (Oct.) 1967.
49. Shimaoka, K., and Sokal, J. E.: Differentiation of benign and malignant thyroid nodules by scintiscan. Arch. Intern. Med. 114:36–39 (July) 1964.
50. Shimkin, P. M., and Sagerman, R. H.: Lymphoma of the thyroid gland. Radiology 92:812–816 (March) 1969.
51. Siber, F. J., and Williams, R. C.: The use of radionuclides for demonstration of pancreatic and hepatic abnormalities. Radiol. Clin. N. Amer. 8:99–113 (April) 1970.
52. Sisson, J. C.: Principles of, and pitfalls in, thyroid function tests. J. Nucl. Med. 6:853–901 (Dec.) 1965.
53. Sodee, D. B.: The evaluation of metastatic thyroid carcinoma with technetium-99m pertechnetate. Radiology 88:145–147 (Jan.) 1967.
54. Strauss, H. W., Hurley, P. J., and Wagner, H. N., Jr.: Advantages of ^{99m}Tc pertechnetate for thyroid scanning in patients with decreased radioiodine uptake. Radiology 97:307–310 (Nov.) 1970.
55. Thomas, C. G., Jr., Pepper, F. D., and Owen, J.: Differentiation of malignant from benign lesions of the thyroid gland using complementary scanning with [75]selenomethionine and radioiodide. Ann. Surg. 170:396–408 (Sept.) 1969.
56. Wagner, H. N. (ed.): Technical details of common procedures. *In* Principles of Nuclear Medicine. Philadelphia, W. B. Saunders Company, 1968, pp. 833–876.
57. Webster, E. W.: Gamma cameras—advantages and disadvantages. Lahey Clin. Found. Bull. 17:67–76 (Jan.-March) 1968.
58. Werner, S. C., and Ingbar, S. H. (eds.): The Thyroid. A Fundamental and Clinical Text. 3rd ed. New York, Harper and Row, 1971.

Chapter Seven

HYPERTHYROIDISM

George O. Bell, M.D.

Hyperthyroidism is a clinical syndrome in which hypermetabolism resulting from excess circulating thyroid hormone is the commonest and most conspicuous manifestation. The total symptom complex includes other important manifestations that are peculiar to one variety of the disease and not to others. Hyperthyroidism occurs in two major forms: toxic diffuse goiter or Graves' disease, and toxic nodular goiter or Plummer's disease.

Factitial hyperthyroidism must always be considered in patients who have hyperthyroidism without goiter or typical eye signs. Less commonly, hyperthyroidism may be part of the early phase of acute or subacute thyroiditis, in which inflammatory changes in the thyroid release excessive amounts of stored hormone into the circulation. Struma ovarii[48] is a rare cause of hyperthyroidism, and carcinoma of the thyroid, even more rarely, may produce hyperthyroidism.

Abnormalities of thyroid function, namely, increase in radioactive iodine uptake, basal metabolic rate, protein-bound iodine, and erythrocyte uptake of triiodothyronine (T3), have been reported in patients with hydatidiform mole and choriocarcinoma.[73] Clinical evidence of thyrotoxicosis is minimal. Odell et al.[74] have demonstrated elevated levels of thyroid-stimulating hormone (TSH) by bioassay in the tumors and plasma from patients with this syndrome. However, radioimmunoassays for pituitary TSH have been negative, indicating that tumor TSH differs from normal human pituitary TSH.

TOXIC DIFFUSE GOITER (GRAVES' DISEASE)

Graves' disease is a constitutional or generalized disease in which hyperthyroidism is only one manifestation. The classic picture includes goiter, hyperthyroidism, exophthalmos, and infiltrative dermopathy (pretibial myxedema), but quite often one or more of these features is absent. Three to 5 percent of patients have no enlargement of the thyroid, although the gland is hyperplastic and its avidity for radioactive iodine is not suppressed by the administration of exogenous thyroid hormone. Hypermetabolism may be the only manifestation of the disease, but sometimes it is minimal or totally absent. Exophthalmos and hyperthyroidism usually occur together and run a parallel course, but at times exophthalmos precedes or follows by many years the hyperthyroid phase. Infiltrative dermopathy usually occurs in association with exophthalmos and is never the sole feature of the disease.

Etiology

The cause of Graves' disease is still unknown. The high familial incidence suggests the possibility of hereditary factors, but as yet no definite pattern of inheritance has been identified.[11, 46] It is likely that more than one genetic aberration exists and, when these are combined with environmental factors, Graves' disease makes its appearance in the patient.[96, 104]

The underlying genetic predisposition to Graves' disease may be activated by various stresses, including emotional trauma, pregnancy, weight reduction, and thyroid hormone therapy.[26, 76] Thyrotoxicosis has appeared following treatment with thyroid hormone and also during hormone therapy when TSH secretion is presumably suppressed.

Pathogenesis

Although the metabolic symptoms of Graves' disease are readily produced in animals and human beings by administration of thyroid hormone, the distinctive ocular and skin changes are always absent, even with large doses. Excessive production of thyroid hormone in Graves' disease is not the primary cause of the syndrome but is merely the factor responsible for hypermetabolism.

Oversecretion of pituitary TSH also is not the primary factor. In fact, excess circulating endogenous thyroid hormone in Graves' disease suppresses pituitary secretion of TSH. Radioimmunoassays of thyrotropin in plasma show absence of circulating TSH.[74, 90] Even though the pituitary-thyroid axis is dormant in Graves' disease, it still remains intact.[65] Myxedema induced by antithyroid drugs activates pituitary TSH secretion, which promptly produces further enlargement of the thyroid. Nonsuppressibility of thyroidal uptake of ^{131}I by administration of thyroid hormone in Graves' disease is further evidence that TSH has no pathogenetic role.[102, 105] If any additional evidence is needed to eliminate TSH as a factor, it is provided by the persistence of typical Graves' disease in hypophysectomized patients who totally lack TSH.[8]

In 1956 Adams and Purves[1, 2] discovered a thyroid-stimulating substance in the serum of patients with Graves' disease. This factor, called long-acting thyroid stimulator (LATS), produces histologic changes in the thyroid characteristic of increased activity. It stimulates both uptake and release of ^{131}I by the thyroid. In contrast to TSH, which causes maximal discharge of ^{131}I from the thyroid gland 2 or 3 hours after injection, LATS induces maximal release of thyroidal radioiodine between 8 and 16 hours after injection. Unfortunately the mouse assay for detection of LATS lacks sufficient sensitivity and reliable quantitation.

LATS activity in serum is detected in only 1 percent of normal subjects and in 9 percent of patients with thyroid disorders other than Graves' disease.[18, 53] When sera have been concentrated, LATS activity has been found in 80 percent of patients with Graves' disease. In thyrotoxic mothers with high serum LATS levels, LATS crosses the placenta and may cause transient hyperthyroidism in newborn babies.[63] Opposed to the above findings, LATS has not been found in the sera of some patients with Graves' disease despite highly concentrated serum techniques and despite active hyperthyroidism or ophthalmopathy. LATS assays are negative in many hyperthyroid patients without ocular changes and even in a number of patients with localized myxedema.

Suppression of serum levels of LATS by corticosteroid therapy originally suggested that LATS might be an antibody.[85] In subsequent studies LATS has been identified as an antibody of the 7S gamma globulin (IgG) variety.[50, 71] It behaves chemically like an IgG immunoglobulin, and its biologic effects can be neutralized by anti-IgG serum but not by anti-TSH serum. The antibody issue is still in doubt, since LATS in the presence of thyroidal antigen gives none of the classic responses of antigen-antibody reaction.[103]

In summary, no proof exists that Graves' disease is caused by autoimmune mechanisms, but evidence suggests that these mechanisms are associated with the disease. Current interest is focused on the possibility that Graves' disease may be an intrinsic or autonomous disorder of the thyroid itself.[90]

Clinical Manifestations of Graves' Disease

The pattern of Graves' disease is quite varied, ranging from very mild to very severe forms with explosive onset and rapid course. The disease occurs in all races and all age groups, but with a high incidence in women. Onset may be abrupt or gradual, covering a period of three to six months. In all cases, the approximate date of onset is easily identified.

Nervous and mental symptoms are prominent and include irritability, emotional lability, restlessness, and activation. A fine tremor of the hands, sometimes not visible, may often be felt by the examiner. In more severe cases the entire body may shake or tremble. Speech is rapid, and responses to questions are instantaneous. Reflexes are hyperactive, and the rapidity of their response is readily seen in the Achilles tendon reflex. Psychoses appearing in patients with severe thyrotoxicosis may require inhospital psychiatric treatment. Correction of the hyperthyroidism is not always followed by equal improvement of the psychoses. Such patients usually have a preexisting abnormal personality structure which decompensates under the stress of thyrotoxicosis.

Cardiovascular symptoms and signs always accompany hyperthyroidism to some degree.[22, 52] They are often ignored or overlooked by young patients but may dominate the picture in the elderly. Thyroid hormone increases myocardial contractility by direct action. Cardiac output is increased, often in excess of total body needs. In mild to moderate thyrotoxicosis, increased heart rate is the primary factor in increasing cardiac output. In severe hyperthyroidism, progressive increase in stroke volume assumes a relatively more important role than increased heart rate in the high cardiac output.

Cardiac action is vigorous, and systolic pressure and pulse pressure are increased. Atrial fibrillation is unusual in patients under the age of 45 and increasingly common in patients over the age of 45. Undoubtedly, occult heart disease exists in some of these patients. However, atrial fibrillation in some thyrotoxic patients may revert to normal sinus rhythm when the euthyroid state is reestablished. Such patients may remain well for years without evidence of any form of heart disease. Persistence of atrial fibrillation after thyrotoxicosis has been cured is not necessarily proof of the existence of underlying heart disease, since many such patients may remain normal indefinitely after normal sinus rhythm is established by drugs or electric shock.

In patients with known heart disease more cardiac symptoms may develop in the presence of hyperthyroidism. Unexplained increase in the frequency and severity of angina pectoris may be the first clue to the existence of hyperthyroidism. Congestive heart failure without underlying independent heart disease is difficult to prove and probably quite rare in thyrotoxicosis, but it is common in those who have preexisting heart disease. Dependent edema, a frequent finding in patients with Graves' disease, is due most often to general vasodilatation and is not in itself evidence of congestive heart failure.

Weight loss in spite of a large appetite is common, but in young persons a weight gain may occur if caloric intake exceeds metabolic demands. In elderly patients, anorexia and severe weight loss are more consistent findings. Increased intestinal motility usually results in more frequent stools but rarely in actual diarrhea.

Muscular weakness and fatigue are prominent.[27] Patients with thigh muscle weakness have difficulty rising from a squatting position, getting up from a low chair, or climbing stairs. Quadriceps weakness is so great at times that patients find it necessary to pull themselves upstairs by their hands or to go upstairs on hands and knees. Generalized muscle wasting usually accompanies severe weight loss. Atrophy of muscles may be seen in the small muscles of the hands, the shoulder girdle, and the temporal muscles. Weakness of the anal sphincter may result in rectal prolapse or fecal incontinence. Occasionally hypokalemic periodic paralysis or myasthenia gravis is associated with Graves' disease.

Gynecomastia,[28] if specifically searched for, is not an uncommon finding. Menstrual cycles are shortened, menstrual flow is decreased, and entire periods may be skipped. Fertility in women with untreated Graves' disease is decreased. All too often conception occurs as hyperthyroidism is being controlled by antithyroid drugs, and the occurrence of pregnancy in the midst of active treatment of Graves' disease presents additional problems.

Heightened metabolism causes increased body warmth and diffuse sweating. Hands and feet are warm; vasodilatation of skin capillaries creates flushing of the face, neck, and upper chest. Thirst is sometimes greatly increased and accompanied by polyuria. Hypercalcemia is occasionally responsible for unusual symptoms.[6, 38]

Physical Findings

Enlargement of the thyroid is usually present and appears with the onset of symptoms or shortly thereafter. The gland is smooth, symmetrical, and diffusely enlarged, but may be irregular if preexisting nodules are present. Some irregularity may be the result of lobulations or congenital variation in the size of the two lobes. In about 5 percent of patients the thyroid is of normal size. Small glands are found most often in elderly patients. A palpable thrill or audible bruit occurs in the large vascular goiters of younger patients.

The eye changes of Graves' disease may be mild, consisting of stare, lid lag, and exophthalmos, or may be severe and characterized by chemosis, edema, mild to moderate protrusion, paralysis of eye muscles, and visual disturbances.[97, 101] The course of ophthalmopathy is unpredictable; it may appear years before the onset of hyperthyroidism or as long as 20 years after the hyperthyroidism has been corrected.[35, 62] More commonly, ocular changes and hyperthyroidism occur within a year or two of each other. Mild eye changes parallel the course of the hyperthyroidism, showing slow improvement when hyperthyroidism has been cured. The infiltrative type of ophthalmopathy tends to follow a course independent of the course of thyrotoxicosis. The benign type of ophthalmopathy may progress to the infiltrative type, and in turn the latter may regress or improve spontaneously.

Pretibial myxedema (infiltrative dermopathy) is never the sole manifestation of Graves' disease; it is almost always accompanied by infiltrative ophthalmopathy. The usual site is the lower third of both legs just above the ankles, but it may also involve the hands, feet, and cheeks. The lesions are bilateral and symmetrical, presenting as small circumscribed lesions or as extensive involvement of the entire lower legs, feet, and toes. The skin is thickened and inelastic. Hair follicles stand out prominently, imparting the appearance of pigskin. In the active phase the color is faintly red or brownish, and lesions feel slightly warm. Aside from the cosmetic problem, localized myxedema is asymptomatic and only rarely causes discomfort or itching.

The thickening and infiltration of the skin is due to deposition of mucopolysaccharides in the dermis and subdermal area similar to the orbital changes in patients with ophthalmopathy. The etiology and pathogenesis are thought to be similar to those of the orbital changes. Localized myxedema pursues a very slow and indolent course, with gradual spread during the active phase, then many months or years without significant change, and finally slow regression of the process. Clubbing of the fingers is occasionally associated with localized myxedema and is possibly a result of the same infiltrative process.

Therapy is rarely necessary. Correction of hyperthyroidism has little if any effect on the skin lesions. Adrenocorticosteroid therapy, at times used in the treatment of the ophthalmopathy, improves the skin lesions, but long-term oral steroid therapy is not justified for treatment of the skin lesions alone. Topical application of steroids, with an occlusive cellophane cover, has helped some patients.[51]

Fingernails are soft, thin, easily broken, and often show peeling of surface layers. The line of attachment of the nail to its bed recedes in an irregular pattern and to a variable degree. Instead of being normally convex, the line is either concave or irregular. The nail changes, often called Plummer's nails, occur only in patients with Graves' disease. Vitiligo, although not specific for Graves' disease, occurs in about 7 percent of patients. It often precedes by many years the occurrence of hyperthyroidism. The distribution of depigmented areas may be widespread but is often localized to the hands and feet, including palms and soles.[72]

The course of untreated Graves' disease is quite variable. Mild cases may subside spontaneously within a year or two. More severe cases persist for years and end fatally in a significant percentage of patients. In a few patients, thyrotoxicosis gradually subsides and is replaced by hypothyroidism. Transition from hyperthyroidism to myxedema can be explained by coexistent inflammatory changes of the Hashimoto's thyroiditis type.[59, 108] Long-term antithyroid drug therapy controls thyrotoxicosis and achieves long-term cure in those patients who have a spontaneous remission.

Differential Diagnosis

The commonest problem in differential diagnosis is presented by the patient with a chronic anxiety state and an incidental goiter. These patients complain of nervousness, irritability, tremor, palpitation, tachycardia, fatigue, insomnia, and sometimes weight loss. Sweating is confined to the face, hands, and axilla and is not generalized. Hands are cold—not warm as in Graves' disease. Other features of Graves' disease are absent. Chronically anxious patients are not immune to the development of Graves' disease, and the diagnosis of the latter must be verified by one or more tests of thyroid function.

Factitial thyrotoxicosis presents the usual symptoms of hypermetabolism but without the typical eye changes, skin changes, or thyroid enlargement. High levels of serum protein-bound iodine (PBI) and serum thyroxine in association with severely depressed 24-hour ^{131}I uptake establish the diagnosis. Identical laboratory results occur in the early phases of acute or subacute thyroiditis, but a greatly elevated sedimentation rate and painful, tender enlargement of the thyroid confirm this diagnosis.

Graves' disease in patients with chronic pulmonary disease, alcoholism, parkinsonism, malignancy, or preexisting heart disease may be concealed by the hypermetabolic symptoms that normally accompany these disorders. Multiple thyroid function tests are needed to verify or eliminate the coexistence of Graves' disease.

Laboratory Tests of Thyroid Function. The multiplicity of thyroid function tests is indeed proof that no single test is specific for the diagnosis of thyroid dysfunction. It is hazardous and misleading to make a diagnosis of hyperthyroidism on the basis of one abnormal test; careful appraisal of the patient's history and physical findings is the foundation for a correct diagnosis. Laboratory tests either support or confirm the clinical impression. The clinician, in turn, must understand the various laboratory tests and know when they are indicated, when they are misleading, and when they are modified by various drugs.

Different tests measure various aspects of thyroid function. The basal metabolic rate is an index of total metabolic effect of thyroid hormone on all body systems. The serum PBI and serum thyroxine are direct measurements of the level of circulating thyroid hormone. Radioiodine uptake measures the thyroid's avidity for iodide. The PBI-131 reflects the output of hormone released from the gland into the circulation. The resin T3 uptake is a measure of thyroxine-binding globulin capacity and indirectly measures the amount of circulating thyroid hormone. Radioiodine uptake before and after 7 to 10 days of T3 ingestion differentiates autonomous goiters such as Graves' disease from compensatory goiters caused by endogenous TSH stimulation. A more detailed analysis of thyroid function tests appears in Chapter Five.

Eye Changes of Graves' Disease

Clinically two separate types of eye changes occur in Graves' disease, one of which is relatively mild, the other severe and often progressive.[97] The mild eye changes consist of stare, lid lag, and proptosis which, from the patient's standpoint, produce few symptoms but constitute a cosmetic problem. The course of this type usually parallels the course of the hyperthyroidism, with gradual though incomplete regression when the thyrotoxic state is controlled. No treatment is required except simple symptomatic measures such as warm compresses, elevation of the head of the bed, and application of artificial tears (methylcellulose eyedrops) at bedtime to avoid corneal drying.

The severe type of ophthalmopathy is characterized by tearing, burning, chemosis, eye muscle weakness, diplopia, periorbital edema, exposure keratitis, corneal ulceration, papilledema, loss of visual acuity and, rarely, panophthalmitis. Proptosis may be slight or moderate, and incomplete closure of eyelids leads to corneal drying with its consequent corneal damage. Progression of the infiltrative process may at times be rapid, creating a serious threat to vision.

The pathologic process is a deposition of water-binding mucopolysaccharides in all tissues of the orbit, including connective tissue, ocular muscles, and eyelids. Tight orbital fascia and ligaments limit the degree of proptosis but lead to greatly increased retro-orbital pressure. Infiltration of the extraocular muscles eventually produces fibrosis, adhesions, and contracture. All muscles are affected, but the inferior rectus and inferior oblique are the most severely involved, resulting in loss of upward movement and sometimes fixation of the globe in a downward position.[56]

The course is erratic and unpredictable. Correction of hyperthyroidism by any method of treatment has no significant effect on the ocular changes.[37, 56, 107] In fact, severe ophthalmopathy not infrequently appears years after the hyperthyroid phase has been cured.[62, 82] Patients who present with both hyperthyroidism and infiltrative ophthalmopathy are treated for their hyperthyroidism in the manner normally indicated for that patient. Antithyroid control prior to thyroidectomy or radioiodine therapy permits observation of the trend of the eye changes. Spontaneous improvement of ophthalmopathy does not occur in the presence of persisting hyperthyroidism. Management of eye changes after correction of hyperthyroidism is determined by their progress.

Severe eye changes require close observation at frequent intervals, usually by an ophthalmologist working with the thyroidologist. Measurement of proptosis, visual acuity tests, and examination of the cornea and fundi, diplopia fields, and visual fields are required to detect any deterioration in the eyes. Corticosteroid therapy in modest doses of 15 to 30 mg. per day may control and relieve moderate symptoms of tearing, pain, chemosis, and early muscle weakness.[15] When the active phase of the process appears to have stabilized, the dose is gradually reduced and finally discontinued. Large doses of prednisone (80 mg. or more per day) are used for treatment of the more ominous developments of papilledema, increasing field defects, decreasing visual acuity, and serious increase in proptosis.[15, 87, 98] The undesirable side effects of long-term steroid therapy are limiting factors. We look on steroid treatment as an extremely valuable method of controlling serious eye problems until the patient can be made euthyroid and ready for orbital decompression.

Surgical decompression of the orbits is indicated primarily to prevent visual loss.[57, 58, 75, 87] Various methods have been advocated by different surgical specialists. At the Lahey Clinic Foundation neurosurgeons have had extensive experience with the intracranial supraorbital approach with very gratifying results. The roof of the orbits is removed as widely as possible to allow maximal upward displacement of the greatly swollen retro-orbital tissues.

Restricted ocular motility and resultant diplopia often persist because of adhesions, fibrosis, and contracture of involved extraocular muscles. Considerable improvement may be afforded by surgical measures. The most frequent operation consists of freeing the inferior rectus from adhesions to the inferior oblique and orbital floor and recessing the inferior rectus an appropriate distance as determined by the experience and judgment of the surgeon.[55]

TOXIC NODULAR GOITER (PLUMMER'S DISEASE)

The process of development of nodular goiter has not yet adequately been explained; many gaps in our knowledge of its etiology remain. Nodular goiter probably has its origin in childhood, particularly at puberty. The primary stimulus appears to be a subnormal level of circulating thyroid hormone secondary to insufficient iodine in food or water, dietary goitrogens which block hormone synthesis, or intrinsic and possibly genetic defects in thyroidal synthesis of hormone. Low levels of circulating thyroid hormone stimulate an increased secretion of pituitary TSH which, in turn, leads to thyroidal hyperplasia and enlargement. Prolonged or intermittent low-grade TSH stimulation causes a change from mild diffuse hyperplasia to a multinodular state. Focal hemorrhage, fibrosis, and calcification result in a fixed or irreversible multinodular goiter which cannot be altered by any form of thyroid suppressive treatment.[66]

Function in the nodules of a multinodular goiter varies from none to moderate or even severe overactivity. Functional activity of the nodules may be enough to suppress function in the remainder of the gland without producing hyperthyroidism, or it may exceed normal hormone requirements and produce hyperthyroidism.[54, 68, 91] There is little or no correlation between the histologic appearance of the nodules and the presence or absence of hyperthyroidism. In glands with hyperfunctioning nodules, the paranodular tissue appears normal or relatively inactive. One or more hyperfunctioning nodules may exist in the same multinodular goiter.

Solitary adenomas are benign encapsulated tumors of the thyroid. These adenomas include papillary, follicular, simple, colloid, or Hürthle cell varieties. Hyperfunction with consequent hyperthyroidism may develop in some patients with discrete adenomas. In 1946 Cope, Rawson, and McArthur[20] defined the entity of hyperfunctioning single adenoma as a cause of thyrotoxicosis. They considered it a rarity, but a 1965 report indicated that solitary toxic autonomous nodules accounted for 13 percent of cases of hyperthyroidism among a group of 537 patients.[54, 91]

In 1956 Boehme et al.[12] reported that scintiscans in 1,015 patients disclosed 74 with hyperfunctioning (hot) nodules associated with partial or complete suppression of the remaining thyroid function. No patient had more than one hyperfunctioning nodule. Cope, Rawson, and McArthur,[20] however, observed two patients with hyperthyroidism associated with two adenomas each. Others have made similar observations. Single hot nodules possess varying degrees of functional activity ranging from euthyroidism to clinical hyperthyroidism. Long-term observations on untreated patients have led to the conclusion that euthyroid hot nodules and toxic nodules represent the same disease in different stages of development. Occasionally, degenerative changes or hemorrhage into a hot nodule destroys its functional activity, leaving instead a nonfunctioning cyst.

A nodular goiter grows in an erratic manner. It gradually enlarges over a period of years, may remain stationary for years, and then may grow again. Some remain small during the life of a patient, whereas others grow to enormous size. A nodular goiter rarely, if ever, disappears spontaneously. Transition from euthyroidism to hyperthyroidism is gradual and insidious, averaging 15 or more years according to Plummer's estimate.[78] Some nodules achieve toxicity within 1 or 2 years, whereas others do so only after 20 to 30 years.

The clinical picture of nodular goiter with hyperthyroidism differs in many ways from that of Graves' disease. The former disease occurs mainly in patients over 40 years of age. The onset is deceptively gradual, requiring several years for full development. Psychic stress is not a precipitating factor. Weight loss is steady, often marked, and usually associated with a poor appetite. Cardiovascular symptoms overshadow the nervous manifestations. Many patients with toxic nodular goiter present a resigned, apathetic outward appearance. The distinctive features of Graves' disease—exophthalmos, pretibial myxedema, and Plummer's nails—do not appear in patients with toxic nodular goiter. Their presence establishes a diagnosis of Graves' disease superimposed on a nodular goiter.

The course of hyperthyroidism caused by nodular goiter is steadily progressive without spontaneous remissions. Therapeutic response to iodides is minimal or lacking, and the response to thiouracil drugs is considerably slower than it is in Graves' disease. Radioiodine therapy is far less effective. Larger doses are required to alleviate the hyperthyroidism, and reduction in goiter size is only minimal. Myxedema following thyroidectomy or radioiodine therapy occurs infrequently. Finally, LATS is absent from the serum of patients with toxic nodular goiter.[64] These differences reinforce the opinion now generally held that toxic nodular goiter and Graves' disease are two distinct entities.

Laboratory Tests

Laboratory tests, with the exception of radioiodine uptake, are generally consistent with the clinical diagnosis. Blackburn and Power[10] found that in patients with toxic nodular goiter 11 percent had PBI levels in the normal range, 22 percent had normal basal metabolic rates, and 57 percent had 24-hour radioiodine uptake in the normal range.[61] We know now that hyperthyroidism in some of these patients is due to an excess production of triiodothyronine rather than thyroxine (T3 thyrotoxicosis).[45, 47, 88, 93] Prolonged administration of thyroxine rarely may suppress ^{131}I uptake in an autonomous nodule, but it fails to decrease the nodule size. Furthermore, thyroid hormone therapy may cause persistent thyrotoxicosis simply by being additive to the hormone produced by the nodule.[67]

In thyroid glands containing a solitary hot nodule, whether toxic or not, 24-hour ^{131}I uptake and scintiscans after a week of T3 administration show little or no change from the initial baseline findings. On the other hand, TSH administration increases the 24-hour radioiodine uptake by stimulating the suppressed nonadenomatous tissue. Together, these two procedures show conclusively that the nodule (or nodules) is autonomous and not under the usual control of endogenous pituitary TSH. Hormone secretion by the nodule is enough to inhibit endogenous TSH secretion, and, in the absence of TSH, the rest of the thyroid gland subsides into a nonfunctioning dormant state. Excision or destruction of the nodule abolishes TSH inhibition, and the nonadenomatous tissue resumes normal function.[54, 91]

TREATMENT OF HYPERTHYROIDISM

The clinician today has a choice of three different methods of treatment of hyperthyroidism, namely, surgery, radioiodine therapy, or long-term therapy with antithyroid drugs. Treatment with each method is directed not toward the primary etiologic agent, which remains unknown, but rather toward the major manifestation of the disease, for example, excessive production of thyroid hormone by an overactive thyroid. In Graves' disease, extrathyroidal features of exophthalmos and pretibial myxedema must be left to pursue their own course, and present-day therapy of these problems is far from satisfactory. In toxic nodular goiter, treatment directed to the thyroid is almost uniformly followed by excellent results.

Selection of a method of treatment in the individual patient is based on the known advantages and disadvantages of the method plus other factors, including availability and skills of the therapist, the physician's own preference, the patient's tolerance of a method of treatment, and the patient's preferences or prejudice. A mode of treatment must be selected which seems most suited to the patient. All three methods of therapy have their place.[42, 57, 77, 86, 100]

Surgical Treatment

Surgical treatment of hyperthyroidism has been in use longer than either radioiodine or long-term antithyroid treatment. When performed by an experienced thyroid surgeon, it restores the patient to a normal euthyroid state more expeditiously and with little risk of mortality or morbidity. The short time span required to achieve cure is a compelling reason favoring its use in selected patients.

Subtotal thyroidectomy is the preferred treatment in patients with toxic nodular goiter, either single or multinodular. It is particularly indicated in patients with large nodular goiters, especially lesions located substernally, either with or without compression of the trachea. Preoperative preparation with antithyroid drugs controls the hyperthyroidism completely, so that thyroidectomy may be performed in a euthyroid patient in a quiet, orderly manner. Although age restrictions for radioiodine therapy in Graves' disease have been lowered or abolished by many thyroidologists, we believe that surgery is preferable for patients in the child-bearing age unless there is a specific contraindication. In children and adolescents, hyperthyroidism is best managed by thyroid surgery. Radioiodine therapy in the young is not justified because of the high incidence of permanent myxedema and the uncertain risks of carcinoma, leukemia, and genetic hazards. If the youthful patient can adapt to long-term medical supervision, a course of antithyroid treatment may be tried first. If relapse occurs after drug therapy is stopped, thyroidectomy is indicated.[30, 77] Thyroidectomy is indicated in patients who are fearful of radiation and who have relapsed after an adequate course of antithyroid drug treatment.

Results of subtotal thyroidectomy performed by skilled and competent surgeons have been good. Mortality is minimal or nil and morbidity is acceptably low.[7, 19] Permanent postoperative tetany is present in less than 0.5 percent, and unilateral vocal cord paralysis in about 0.5 percent; hyperthyroidism recurs in approximately 3 percent. Postoperative myxedema based on a five-year follow-up occurs in 5 to 10 percent of patients. In longer follow-up studies, postoperative myxedema is found in up to 40 percent of patients. After the first postoperative year the increment in myxedema is 1.7 percent per year.[70] Mild degrees of subnormal thyroid function that would be missed if only clinical signs were used in making the diagnosis of hypothyroidism are detected by T4 and TSH determinations. Thus, the incidence of postoperative hypothyroidism has shown an apparent increase. Periodic follow-up examinations must be considered an essential part of the therapeutic program.

The major advantage of surgery is the rapidity with which the patient is relieved of hyperthyroidism and restored to a euthyroid state. In this sense surgery is more predictable and definitive, and the patient resumes his normal living pattern in a matter of eight to ten weeks. Exacerbation in the ophthalmopathy following thyroidectomy in Graves' disease has been overemphasized. Although a small increase in eye protrusion may occur after surgery, progression of major infiltrative eye changes seems independent of the therapy directed toward the thyroid. Progression may occur after any form of therapy, including surgery, radioiodine, and antithyroid treatment. On the other hand, spontaneous regression of ophthalmic findings has not occurred in the presence of persisting hyperthyroidism. Correction of thyrotoxicosis has been followed by gradual improvement in eye changes in many patients. During the preoperative preparation with antithyroid drugs, the eye changes may be observed closely. The doctor gains the patient's confidence and educates him in the variable behavior of ocular problems. When the ophthalmopathy stabilizes, thyroidectomy may be performed.

Radioiodine Treatment

Treatment of Graves' disease with radioactive iodine was first reported in 1942.[36, 44] In 1946, ^{131}I was made available for general use, and since then many thousands of thyrotoxic patients have been treated by this agent. The special capacity of the thyroid to accumulate and concentrate iodine within the thyroid cells makes it possible to deposit a radiation dose directly into the gland. That portion of the dose of ^{131}I not retained by the hyperplastic gland is quickly eliminated from the body, mainly by the kidneys. Thus, the thyroid gland is selectively radiated. Radiation of the thyroid gland obtains its therapeutic effect by destruction of some thyroid cells, injury to the genetic mechanism for cell division, and impairment of thyroid cell function. Histologic changes in the thyroid include cellular necrosis, nuclear changes, fibrosis, and blood vessel changes.[100] Radioiodine therapy is, in effect, a medical thyroidectomy. If an ideal dose is administered, the patient returns to a euthyroid state and the thyroid returns to normal size. Should the dose of ^{131}I be too small, hyperthyroidism persists, and if too large, hypothyroidism develops relatively soon after the therapy.

Radioiodine is universally accepted as the preferred treatment for patients with Graves' disease recurring after previous surgery, Graves' disease in patients more than 40 years of age, and Graves' disease complicated by other major diseases which increase the risk of anesthesia and surgery. Many thyroid centers have lowered the age limit to 25 years, and a few centers treat patients of all ages with ^{131}I. More conservative thyroidologists avoid the use of radioiodine in children and in young adults in the child-bearing years. This approach coincides with our own philosophy, although other factors of importance may modify this position. Toxic nodular goiter is more effectively treated surgically. Radioiodine therapy is used only when the surgical risk is prohibitive. The dose of radioiodine required to effect a cure is two or more times the dose needed in Graves' disease, and the possibility of permanent cure is less certain.

Pregnancy is the absolute contraindication to radioiodine therapy, and almost of equal importance as a contraindication is the patient's fear of radiation. Unless the patient willingly accepts radioiodine therapy, this form of treatment should be avoided. All symptoms appearing subsequent to treatment will be attributed rightly or wrongly to the radioiodine. It is difficult to convince the patient that a carcinoma of the cervix, breast, or elsewhere, appearing within a year after radioiodine therapy, was not caused by the radiation. Finally, radioiodine is not selected for treatment if findings in the thyroid suggest the possibility of malignancy. Relative contraindications to ^{131}I therapy include Graves' disease in children and toxic multinodular goiters.

A major problem of radioiodine therapy is the selection of the minimal effective dose that cures the hyperthyroidism without undue delay and without producing myxedema.[33, 34] Fears of possible carcinogenesis and of leukemia have been eliminated by the U.S. Public Health study of patients treated in the past, which failed to find a significantly increased frequency of leukemia[81] or thyroid cancer[24] in hyperthyroid patients treated with radioiodine compared to patients treated surgically.

Methods for calculating the dose of ^{131}I in patients with Graves' disease vary from specific formulas to pure random choice,[79, 84] and results of therapy have ben remarkably similar. Most methods attempt to quantitate the dose in relation to the estimated size of the goiter—an estimation which even in experienced hands may be inaccurate. Factors other than thyroid size are important determinants in the effectiveness of a therapeutic dose of radioiodine. These include the uniformity of distribution of the isotope within the gland, the amount accumulated by the thyroid, the effective half-life, and the sensitivity of the thyroid cells to radiation. This last factor is totally unpredictable and yet has significant influence on the final outcome of treatment.

A common practice in radioiodine therapy is to administer a dose of 150 to 160 μCi. of ^{131}I per estimated gram of thyroid. If the previously determined 24-hour thyroidal uptake is below 75 percent, the dose is increased appropriately. To calculate the dose based on actual 24-hour uptake, the following formula may be used:[79]

$$\text{Dose of } ^{131}\text{I} = \frac{\text{Estimated thyroid weight in grams} \times 150}{\text{24-hour }^{131}\text{I uptake}}$$

For a 40-gm. goiter with an uptake of 60 percent, the dose of ^{131}I is $\frac{40 \times 150}{0.60} = 10,000$ μCi. or 10 mCi.

Permanent myxedema has emerged as a major complication following radioactive iodine therapy. Dunn and Chapman[25] reported an incidence of myxedema of 20 percent within two years after treatment, with a yearly increment of 2 to 3 percent with continued follow-up. At the end of 10 years 43 percent of patients had permanent myxedema.

Other reports indicate an incidence of myxedema of 30 to 70 percent after 10 years.[14, 29]

In an effort to reduce the high incidence of myxedema after treatment, reduction of the initial dose of radioiodine to 80 μCi. per gram of thyroid tissue has been suggested.[33, 34] In many patients so treated there has been a cure of the thyrotoxicosis and a lower incidence of myxedema. The follow-up period has not been long enough to evaluate the long-term effects. Response of thyrotoxicosis to the reduced dose of ^{131}I has been delayed in many patients, so that persistent hyperthyroidism, if moderate or severe, must be treated with additional doses of radioiodine. Persistent hyperthyroidism, if mild, may be controlled by administration of potassium iodide maintained over a period of months until the long-term effect of radiation has become clearly established. Failure of the goiter to decrease in size during this time usually indicates that hyperthyroidism will persist.

Long-term Antithyroid Treatment

Since 1943 when Astwood[5] introduced thiouracil as a treatment of hyperthyroidism, drug treatment of this disease has been extensive. Accumulated experience has established long-term drug therapy as an effective form of treatment in selected patients.

The thiocarbamides, propylthiouracil and methimazole (Tapazole) are used most frequently in this country, whereas carbimazole (Neomercazole) is preferred in Europe. They are less toxic than the original thiouracil and fully as effective. They inhibit thyroid hormone formation by interference with oxidation of the iodide ion, its binding to tyrosine, and the coupling of iodotyrosines into T3 and thyroxine (T4). They also inhibit the conversion of MIT to DIT and, in the case of propylthiouracil, the peripheral deiodination of thyroxine.[92] They are rapidly absorbed from the intestine, have a prompt effect on the thyroid as measured by thyroidal accumulation of ^{131}I, and a moderately rapid decline in its effect.[86] Effective blocking of hormone formation requires spacing of daily doses at six- to eight-hour intervals. This is important in the severely toxic patient, but less so in mildly toxic patients, who respond satisfactorily to doses at 12- or even 24-hour intervals.[31]

Prolonged antithyroid treatment is indicated in patients under 40 years of age with mild to moderately severe Graves' disease of recent onset or short duration with relatively small goiters (50 gm. or less). The patient must be dependable, cooperative, and available for long-term observation. Opinion is divided as to whether long-term drug treatment or thyroidectomy after short-term preparation is preferred for children[39, 40, 49] and adolescents and for pregnant women.[9, 13, 41, 99] Both methods have given satisfactory results. The severity of thyrotoxicity and the ease with which it is controlled by antithyroid drugs are major factors in selection of treatment for pregnant patients. Children and adolescents who have relapses after adequate long-term antithyroid treatment are best treated with thyroid surgery. Long-term drug therapy is not indicated in patients with toxic nodular goiter unless the goiter is nonobstructive and surgical risk is prohibitive.

The usual plan for long-term medical therapy consists of the administration of 300 to 750 mg. of propylthiouracil or 30 to 60 mg. of methimazole daily in three or four divided doses.[43, 80, 106] When a euthyroid state is reached, the dose is gradually reduced to a maintenance level sufficient to hold the patient at the euthyroid level. Desiccated thyroid (120 to 180 mg. daily) is added to avoid the inadvertent occurrence of hypothyroidism and at the same time permit a dose of antithyroid drug large enough to control thyrotoxicity completely. The euthyroid state is maintained for at least 12 months, at which time the dosage of the antithyroid drug is gradually reduced and finally stopped. Administration of desiccated thyroid alone is continued for several months, during which time a 24-hour radioactive iodine uptake is performed. If uptake is suppressed below 20 percent, permanent remission is likely. Nonsuppression of uptake is strong evidence that clinical relapse will follow.[3, 17]

The major disadvantage of long-term medical therapy is the unpredictability of a successful outcome. Permanent remissions occur in only 50 to 55 percent of patients. Most relapses (60 to 70 percent) occur within the first year after completion of treatment. The one clue pointing to possible remission is a decrease in the size of the goiter, but unfortunately this is usually delayed until late in the course of therapy. The 20-minute uptake of ^{131}I determined at intervals while the patient is taking antithyroid drug and thyroid hormone, as reported by Alexander et al.,[3] may provide an earlier indication of possible remission. Patients who demonstrate suppression of uptake within the first six months are most likely to achieve a lasting remission after the full course of treatment. Patients with negative suppression tests at six months usually have relapses shortly after medical treatment is stopped. If the reliability of the suppression test is verified by further experience, patients with nonsuppressible uptakes at six months can promptly be advised to have definitive treatment with radioiodine or surgery.

Toxic reactions to propylthiouracil or methimazole occur in 3 to 5 percent of patients. Drug fever, skin rashes, nausea, vomiting, diarrhea, arthralgias, hepatitis, and bone marrow depression may occur. Leukopenia, thrombocytopenia, and agranulocytosis are all possible. The incidence of agranulocytosis is 0.3 percent.[86] Fatalities may occur but usually can be prevented by early and adequate treatment. Patients who have adverse reactions to one drug may tolerate the other; those who react adversely to both drugs are treated with either radioiodine or thyroidectomy. Failure of the patient to comply with the prescribed program of drug treatment reduces the chances of achieving a permanent remission. In such cases, an alternative treatment plan should be instituted without delay.

THYROID CRISIS OR STORM

Thyroid storm is a severe exacerbation of the hyperthyroid state, usually of sudden onset and frequently ending fatally. Mortality rate during the iodine era was 60 to 70 percent or higher, but with current methods of treatment it has been reduced to around 25 percent. In the past, thyroid storm most frequently followed thyroid surgery but, with antithyroid drug preparation, postoperative storms have been virtually eliminated. Now most instances of thyroid storms are precipitated by intercurrent infection, surgical procedures other than on the thyroid, diabetic keto-acidosis, trauma, or other severe stresses which occur at times when thyrotoxicosis is either untreated or only partially controlled by antithyroid therapy.[60, 69, 94]

Thyroid storm is manifested by marked increase in hyperthyroidism, fever as high as 103 to 106° F. (39.4 to 41.1° C.), severe tachycardia, and evidence of critical dysfunction in the central nervous, cardiovascular, and gastrointestinal systems, including the liver. Restlessness, severe agitation, mental confusion, hallucinations, and frank psychosis are common, but in some patients somnolence, apathy, severe muscular weakness, and coma are predominant. Severe tachycardia, auricular fibrillation, and congestive heart failure may occur. Vomiting, diarrhea, and jaundice added to the pyrexia often lead to severe dehydration and electrolyte imbalance. Superimposed symptoms associated with the precipitating cause exaggerate and modify the total picture.

Laboratory findings during a crisis have necessarily been limited because of the critical state of the patient. The results of the usual tests of thyroid function are elevated. The protein-bound iodine level has varied, depending on the amount of previous antithyroid treatment. Protein-bound iodine levels are commonly in a range of 11 to 15 μg. per 100 ml., but occasionally are well over 20 μg. per 100 ml. Other laboratory tests reflect abnormalities induced by the intercurrent pathologic process.

Treatment

Prevention of thyroid storm is a major objective in the management of all patients with hyperthyroidism. Thyroid surgery must be withheld until complete control of hyperthyroidism by antithyroid preparation is achieved. Thyroidectomy in the presence of even mild degrees of hyperthyroidism may precipitate a postoperative storm, particularly in Graves' disease. Surgery other than on the thyroid gland should be delayed when possible until euthyroidism has been achieved by antithyroid treatment. When delay is impossible or hazardous, treatment for storm should be started and continued until the patient has passed the critical stress.

The first therapeutic move in treatment of storm is to block hormone formation by propylthiouracil or methimazole and block release of hormone from the thyroid by iodides. Propylthiouracil is given by mouth or by stomach tube in doses of 250 to 500 mg. at six-hour intervals. Sodium iodide is given intravenously in doses of 1 to 3 gm. a day. It is important that propylthiouracil block to hormone synthesis is instituted before iodides are administered to prevent the incorporation of iodides into more hormone. Hydrocortisone is administered intravenously in doses of 100 mg. every eight hours. If infection is present or even suspected as a precipitating factor, antibiotics are given. Treatment is initiated with a broad-spectrum antibiotic until bacteriologic studies are available. Either reserpine,[16, 23, 69, 94] 2.5 mg. intramuscularly every 8 hours, or guanethidine,[23, 60, 69, 95] 50 mg. orally or intramuscularly every 12 hours, is used for its sympatholytic effect. Reserpine is preferred for the agitated patient because of its sedative effect; guanethidine is preferred in somnolent or apathetic patients. With either drug the dose is titrated according to the patient's response, particularly heart rate, blood pressure, and mental picture.

Sympathetic blockade with propranolol (beta adrenergic blocking agent) alone[21, 32, 83] or with a combination of propranolol and phenoxybenzamine hydrochloride (specific alpha blocking agent)[89] has been recommended as adjuvant treatment for patients with severe thyrotoxicosis. The recommended oral dose of propranolol is 80 to 120 mg. four times a day, and phenoxybenzamine hydrochloride 10 mg. two to four times daily. Experience with these agents has not been sufficiently extensive to assess their proper place in the therapeutic regimen.

Other supportive therapy includes replacement of fluids and electrolytes, control of fever with aspirin, alcohol sponging or ice mattress, oxygen, digitalis for congestive heart failure, and large doses of B complex vitamins. Plasmaphoresis has been used effectively to reduce serum thyroxine levels in patients not responding well to the above measures.[4]

The duration of the storm varies from one to eight days. Patients responding favorably usually recover within 72 hours. Fatalities will occur even with the best management. Thyroid storm is a devastating complication of hyperthyroidism but, fortunately, it is rare.

REFERENCES

1. Adams, D. D.: The presence of an abnormal thyroid-stimulating hormone in the serum of some thyrotoxic patients. J. Clin. Endocr. 18:699–712 (July) 1958.
2. Adams, D. D., and Purves, H. D.: Abnormal responses in the assay of thyrotrophin. Proc. Univ. Otago Medical School 34:11–12 (April) 1956.
3. Alexander, W. D., Harden, R. M., Shimmins, J., et al.: Treatment of thyrotoxicosis based on thyroidal suppressibility. Lancet 2:681–684 (Sept. 30) 1967.
4. Ashkar, F. S., Katims, R. B., Smoak, W. M., 3d, et al.: Thyroid storm treatment with blood exchange and plasmapheresis. J.A.M.A. 214:1275–1279 (Nov. 16) 1970.
5. Astwood, E. B.: Treatment of hyperthyroidism with thiourea and thiouracil. J.A.M.A. 122:78–81 (May 8) 1943.
6. Baxter, J. D., and Bondy, P. K.: Hypercalcemia of thyrotoxicosis. Ann. Intern. Med. 65:429–442 (Sept.) 1966.
7. Beahrs, O. H., and Sakulsky, S. B.: Surgical thyroidectomy in the management of exophthalmic goiter. Arch. Surg. 96:512–516 (April) 1968.

8. Becker, D. V., and Furth, E. D.: Total surgical hypophysectomy in nine patients with Graves' disease: Evidence for extra-pituitary maintenance of this disorder. In Cassano, C. E., and Andreoli, M. (eds.): Current Topics in Thyroid Research. Proceedings of Fifth International Thyroid Conference, Rome, 1965. New York, Academic Press, 1965, pp. 596–602.
9. Bell, G. O., and Hall, J.: Hyperthyroidism in pregnancy. Med. Clin. N. Amer. 44:363–367 (March) 1960.
10. Blackburn, C. M., and Power, M. H.: Diagnostic accuracy of serum protein-bound iodine determination in thyroid disease. J. Clin. Endocr. 15:1379–1392 (Nov.) 1955.
11. Boas, N. F., and Ober, W. B.: Hereditary exophthalmic goitre—report of eleven cases in one family. J. Clin. Endocr. 6:575–588 (Aug.) 1946.
12. Boehme, E. J., Kugel, A., Specht, N., et al.: The thyroid scintigram: An evaluation of its clinical use. Trans. Amer. Goiter Ass., (May) 1956, pp. 422–433.
13. Bokat, M. A.: Treatment of hyperthyroidism during pregnancy. In Astwood, E. B., and Cassidy, C. E. (eds.): Clinical Endocrinology. Vol. 2. New York, Grune & Stratton, 1968, pp. 236–243.
14. Bronsky, D., Kiamko, R. T., and Walstein, S. S.: Post-therapeutic myxedema. Relative occurrence after treatment of hyperthyroidism by radioactive iodine (131-I) or subtotal thyroidectomy. Arch. Intern. Med. 121:113–117 (Feb.) 1968.
15. Brown, J., Coburn, J. W., Wigod, R. A., et al.: Adrenal steroid therapy of severe infiltrative ophthalmopathy of Graves' disease. Amer. J. Med. 34:786–795 (June) 1963.
16. Canary, J. J., Schaaf, M., Duffy, B. J., Jr., et al.: Effects of oral and intramuscular administration of reserpine in thyrotoxicosis. New Engl. J. Med. 257:435–442 (Sept. 5) 1957.
17. Cassidy, C. E.: Use of a thyroid suppression test as a guide to prognosis of hyperthyroidism treated with antithyroid drugs. J. Clin. Endocr. 25:155–156 (Feb.) 1965.
18. Chopra, I. J., and Solomon, D. H.: The thyroid gland in Graves' disease: Victim or culprit? J. Clin. Invest. 49:18a–19a 1970. (Supplement.)
19. Colcock, B. P., and King, M. L.: The mortality and morbidity of thyroid surgery. Surg. Gynec. Obstet. 114:131–136 (Feb.) 1962.
20. Cope, O., Rawson, R. W., and McArthur, J. W.: Hyperfunctioning single adenoma of thyroid. Surg. Gynec. Obstet. 84:415–426 (April) 1947.
21. Das, G., and Krieger, M.: Treatment of thyrotoxic storm with intravenous administration of propranolol. Ann. Intern. Med. 70:985–988 (May) 1969.
22. DeGroot, L. J., and Leonard, J. J.: Hyperthyroidism as a high cardiac output state. Amer. Heart J. 79:265–275 (Feb.) 1970.
23. Dillon, P. T., Babe, J., Meloni, C. R., et al.: Reserpine in thyrotoxic crisis. New Engl. J. Med. 283:1020–1023 (Nov. 5) 1970.
24. Dobyns, B. M., Sheline, G. E., Workman, J. B., et al.: Incidence of benign and malignant lesions of the thyroid in patients treated for hyperthyroidism. A Report of the Cooperative Thyrotoxicosis Therapy Follow-up Study. In Program of the 1969 Meeting of the American Thyroid Association, Chicago, Illinois, p. 52.
25. Dunn, J. T., and Chapman, E. M.: Rising incidence of hypothyroidism after radioactive-iodine therapy in thyrotoxicosis. New Engl. J. Med. 271:1037–1042 (Nov. 12) 1964.
26. Dymling, J. F., and Becker, D. V.: Occurrence of hyperthyroidism in patients receiving thyroid hormone. J. Clin. Endocr. 27:1487–1491 (Oct.) 1967.
27. Engel, A. G.: Neuromuscular manifestations of Graves' disease. Mayo Clin. Proc. 47:919–925 (Dec.) 1972.
28. Gorman, C. A.: Unusual manifestations of Graves' disease. Mayo Clin. Proc. 47:926–933 (Dec.) 1972.
29. Green, M., and Wilson, G. M.: Thyrotoxicosis treated by surgery or iodine-131. With special reference to development of hypothyroidism. Brit. Med. J. 1:1005–1010 (April) 1964.
30. Green, W., and Wessler, S.: Management of juvenile hyperthyroidism. J.A.M.A. 213:1652–1655 (Sept. 7) 1970.
31. Greer, M. A., Meihoff, W. C., and Studer, H.: Treatment of hyperthyroidism with a single daily dose of propylthiouracil. New Engl. J. Med. 272:888–891 (April 29) 1965.

32. Hadden, D. R., Montgomery, D. A., Shanks, R. G., et al.: Propranolol and iodine-131 in the management of thyrotoxicosis. Lancet 2:852–854 (Oct. 19) 1968.
33. Hagen, G. A.: Treatment of thyrotoxicosis with 131-I and post-therapy hypothyroidism. Med. Clin. N. Amer. 52:417–429 (March) 1968.
34. Hagen, G. S., Ouellette, R. P., and Chapman, E. M.: Comparison of high and low dosage levels of 131-I in the treatment of thyrotoxicosis. New Engl. J. Med. 277:559–562 (Sept. 14) 1967.
35. Hamilton, H. E., Schultz, R. O., and DeGowin, E. L.: The endocrine eye lesions in hyperthyroidism: Its incidence and course in 165 patients treated for thyrotoxicosis with iodine. Arch. Intern. Med. 105:675–685 (May) 1960.
36. Hamilton, J. G., and Lawrence, J. H.: Recent clinical developments in the therapeutic application of radio-phosphorus and radio-iodine. J. Clin. Invest. 21:624 (Sept.) 1942.
37. Hamilton, R. D., Mayberry, W. E., McConahey, W. M., et al.: Ophthalmopathy of Graves' disease: A comparison between patients treated surgically and patients treated with radioiodide. Mayo Clin. Proc. 42:812–818 (Dec.) 1967.
38. Harper, P. S., and Hughes, R. O.: Severe hypercalcemia from hyperthyroidism with unusual features. Brit. Med. J. 1:213–214 (Jan. 24) 1970.
39. Hayles, A. B., and Chaves-Carballo, E.: Exophthalmic goiter in children: A therapeutic trial with antithyroid drugs. Mayo Clin. Proc. 40:889–894 (Dec.) 1965.
40. Hayles, A. B., Chaves-Carballo, E., and McConahey, W. M.: The treatment of hyperthyroidism (Graves' disease) in children. Mayo Clin. Proc. 42:218–224 (April) 1967.
41. Herbst, A. L., and Selenkow, H. A.: Hyperthyroidism during pregnancy. New Engl. J. Med. 273:627–633 (Sept. 16) 1965.
42. Hershman, J. M.: Treatment of hyperthyroidism. Mod. Treat. 6:497–515 (May) 1969.
43. Hershman, J. M., Givens, J. R., Cassidy, C. E., et al.: Long-term outcome of hyperthyroidism treated with antithyroid drugs. J. Clin. Endocr. 26:803–807 (Aug.) 1966.
44. Hertz, S., and Roberts, A.: Application of radioactive iodine in therapy of Graves' disease. J. Clin. Invest. 21:624 (Sept.) 1942.
45. Hollander, C. S., Mitsuma, T., Nihei, N., et al.: Clinical and laboratory observations in cases of triiodothyronine toxicosis confirmed by radioimmunoassay. Lancet 1:609–611 (March 18) 1972.
46. Ingbar, S. H., Freinkel, N., Dowling, J. T., et al.: Abnormalities of iodine metabolism in euthyroid relatives of patients with Graves' disease. J. Clin. Invest. 35:714 (June) 1956.
47. Ivy, H. K., Wahner, H. W., and Gorman, C. A.: Triiodothyronine (T3) toxicosis. Its role in Graves' disease. Arch. Intern. Med. 128:529–534 (Oct.) 1971.
48. Kempers, R. D., Dockerty, M. B., Hoffman, D. L., et al.: Struma ovarii—ascitic, hyperthyroid, and asymptomatic syndromes. Ann. Intern. Med. 72:883–893 (June) 1970.
49. Kogut, M. D., Kaplan, S. A., Collipp, P. J., et al.: Treatment of hyperthyroidism in children. Analysis of forty-five patients. New. Engl. J. Med. 272:217–221 (Feb. 4) 1965.
50. Kriss, J. P., Pleshakov, V., and Chien, J. R.: Isolation and identification of long-acting thyroid stimulator and its relation to hyperthyroidism and circumscribed pretibial myxedema. J. Clin. Endocr. 24:1005–1028 (Oct.) 1964.
51. Kriss, J. P., Pleshakov, V., Rosenblum. A., et al.: Therapy with occlusive dressings of pretibital myxedema with fluocinolone acetonide. J. Clin. Endocr. 27:595–604 (May) 1967.
52. Leonard, J. J., and DeGroot, L. J.: The thyroid state and the cardiovascular system. Mod. Conc. Cardiovasc. Dis. 38:23–27 (May) 1969.
53. Lipman, L. M., Green, D. E., Snyder, N. J., et al.: Relationship of long-acting thyroid stimulator to the clinical features and course of Graves' disease. Amer. J. Med. 43:486–498 (Oct.) 1967.
54. Lobo, L. C. G., Rosenthal, D., and Fridman, J.: Evolution of autonomous thyroid nodules. In Cassano, C. E., and Andreoli, M. (eds.): Current Topics in Thyroid Research. Proceedings of Fifth International Thyroid Conference, Rome, 1965. New York, Academic Press, 1965, pp. 892–899.
55. Long, J. C.: Surgical management of tropias of thyroid exophthalmos. Arch. Ophthal. 75:634–638 (May) 1966.

56. Long, J. C.: Medical and Surgical Management of Endocrine Exophthalmos. 1969 Instruction Section, Course 220. American Academy of Ophthalmology and Otolaryngology, 15 Second St. SW, Rochester, Minn 55901.
57. Long, J. C., and Ellis, G. D.: Temporal decompression of the orbit for thyroid exophthalmos. Amer. J. Ophthal. 62:1089–1098 (Dec.) 1966.
58. MacCarty, C. S., Kenefick, T. P., McConahey, W. M., et al.: Ophthalmopathy of Graves' disease treated by removal of roof, lateral walls and lateral sphenoid ridge: Review of 46 cases. Mayo Clin. Proc. 45:488–493 (July) 1970.
59. Mason, R. E., and Walsh, F. B.: Exophthalmos in hypothyroidism due to Hashimoto's thyroiditis. Bull. Johns Hopkins Hosp. 112:323–329 (June) 1963.
60. Mazzaferri, E. L., and Skillman, T. G.: Thyroid storm. A review of 22 episodes with special emphasis on the use of guanethidine. Arch. Intern. Med. 124:684–690 (Dec.) 1969.
61. McConahey, W. M., Owen, C. A., Jr., and Keating, F. R., Jr.: Clinical appraisal of radioiodine tests of thyroid function. J. Clin. Endocr. 16:724–734 (June) 1956.
62. McHugh, J. J., and Mellinger, R. C.: Progressive exophthalmos developing 12 years after thyroidectomy for diffuse toxic goiter. Ann. Intern. Med. 49:955–958 (Oct.) 1958.
63. McKenzie, J. M.: Neonatal Graves' disease. J. Clin. Endocr. 24:660–668 (July) 1964.
64. McKenzie, J. M.: Hyperthyroidism caused by thyroid adenomata. J. Clin. Endocr. 26:779–781 (July) 1966.
65. Means, J. H., DeGroot, L. J., and Stanbury, J. B.: The Thyroid and Its Diseases. Ed. 3. New York, McGraw-Hill Book Company, Inc., 1963, p. 168.
66. Meissner, W. A., and Warren, S.: Tumors of the thyroid gland. Atlas of Tumor Pathology, Second Series, Fascicle 4. Washington, D.C., Armed Forces Institute of Pathology, 1969.
67. Miller, J. M., and Block, M. A.: Functional autonomy in multinodular goiter. J.A.M.A. 214:535–539 (Oct. 19) 1970.
68. Miller, J. M., Horn, R. C., and Block, M. A.: The autonomous functioning thyroid nodule in the evolution of nodular goiter. J. Clin. Endocr. 27:1264–1274 (Sept.) 1967.
69. Nelson, N. C., and Becker, W. F.: Thyroid crisis: Diagnosis and treatment. Ann. Surg. 170:263–273 (Aug.) 1969.
70. Nofal, M. M., Beierwaltes, W. H., and Patno, M. E.: Treatment of hyperthyroidism with sodium iodide I-131. J.A.M.A. 197:605–610 (Aug. 22) 1966.
71. Ochi, Y., and DeGroot, L. J.: Long acting thyroid stimulator of Graves' disease. New Engl. J. Med. 278:718–721 (March 28) 1968.
72. Ochi, Y., and DeGroot, L. J.: Vitiligo in Graves' disease. Ann. Intern. Med. 71:935–940 (Nov.) 1969.
73. Odell, W. D., Bates, R. W., Rivlin, R. S., et al.: Increased thyroid function without clinical hyperthyroidism in patients with choriocarcinoma. J. Clin. Endocr. 23:658–664 (July) 1963.
74. Odell, W. D., Wilber, J. F., and Paul, W. E.: Radioimmunoassay of human thyrotropin in serum. Metabolism 14:465–467 (April) 1965.
75. Ogura, J. H.: Transantral orbital decompression for progressive exophthalmos. A follow-up of 54 cases. Med. Clin. N. Amer. 52:399–407 (March) 1968.
76. Paz, A. T., Zellmann, H. E., and Bell, G. O.: Graves' disease following thyroid therapy. Lahey Clin. Found. Bull. 18:11–16 (Jan.-March) 1969.
77. Pittman, J. A., Jr., and Pittman, C. S.: Treatment of hyperthyroidism. GP 31:137–144 (April) 1965.
78. Plummer, H. S.: The clinical and pathologic relationships of hyperplastic and non-hyperplastic goiter. J.A.M.A. 61:650–651 (Aug. 30) 1913.
79. Rawson, R. W., Money, W. L., and Grief, R. L.: Diseases of the thyroid. *In* Bondy, P. K., and Rosenberg, L. E. (eds.): Duncan's Diseases of Metabolism. Ed. 6. Philadelphia, W. B. Saunders Co., 1969, p. 798.
80. Reveno, W. S., and Rosenbaum, H.: Observations on the use of antithyroid drugs. Ann. Intern. Med. 60:982–989 (June) 1964.
81. Saenger, E. L., Thoma, G. E., and Thompkins, E. A.: Incidence of leukemia following treatment of hyperthyroidism. Preliminary Report of the Cooperative Thyrotoxicosis Therapy Follow-up Study. J.A.M.A. 205:855–862 (Sept. 16) 1968.
82. Scholz, D. A., Haines, S. F., and Henderson, J. W.: Ophthalmopathy associated with Graves' disease. Unusual clinical manifestations and their management. Arch. Intern. Med. 109:526–535 (May) 1962.

83. Shanks, R. D., Hadden, R. D., Lowe, D. C., et al.: Controlled trial of propranolol in thyrotoxicosis. Lancet 1:993–994 (May 17) 1969.
84. Skillman, T. G., Mazzaferri, E. L., and Gwinup, G.: Random dosage of 131-I in the treatment of hyperthyroidism: results of a prospective study. Amer. J. Med. Sci. 257:382–387 (June) 1969.
85. Snyder, N. J., Green, D. E., and Solomon, D. H.: Glucocorticoid-induced disappearance of long-acting thyroid stimulator in the ophthalmopathy of Graves' disease. J. Clin. Endocr. 24:1129–1135 (Nov) 1964.
86. Solomon, D. H. (Moderator): Hyperthyroidism. U.C.L.A. Interdepartmental Conference. Ann. Intern. Med. 69:1015–1035 (Nov.) 1968.
87. Solomon, D. H.: Treatment of extrathyroidal manifestations of Graves' disease. Mod. Treat. 6:516–533 (May) 1969.
88. Sterling, K., Refetoff, S., and Selenkow, H. A.: T3 thyrotoxicosis. Thyrotoxicosis due to elevated serum triiodythyronine levels. J.A.M.A. 213:571–575 (July 27) 1970.
89. Stout, B. D., Wiener, L., and Cox, J. W.: Combined alpha and beta sympathetic blockade in hyperthyroidism. Clinical and metabolic effects. Ann. Intern. Med. 70:963–970 (May) 1970.
90. Utiger, R. D.: Immunoassay of human plasma TSH. In Cassano, C. E., and Andreoli, M. (eds.): Current Topics in Thyroid Research. Proceedings of Fifth International Thyroid Conference, Rome, 1965. New York, Academic Press, 1965, pp. 513–526.
91. Vague, J., Simonin, R., Miller, G., et al.: Diagnosis and evolution of autonomous secreting thyroid nodules. In Cassano, C. E., and Andreoli, M. (eds.): Current Topics in Thyroid Research. Proceedings of Fifth International Thyroid Conference. Rome, 1965. New York, Academic Press, 1965, pp. 883–891.
92. Vanderlaan, W. P.: Antithyroid drugs in practice. Mayo Clin. Proc. 47:962–965 (Dec.) 1972.
93. Wahner, H. W.: T3 hyperthyroidism. Mayo Clin. Proc. 47:938–943 (Dec.) 1972.
94. Waldstein, S. S., Slodki, S. J., Kaganiec, I., et al.: A clinical study of thyroid storm. Ann. Intern. Med. 52:626–642 (March) 1960.
95. Waldstein, S. S., West, G. H., Jr., Lee, W. Y., et al.: Guanethidine in hyperthyroidism. J.A.M.A. 189:609–612 (Aug. 24) 1964.
96. Weinstein, B., and Kitchin, F. D.: In Werner, S. C., and Ingbar, S. H. (eds.): The Thyroid. Ed. 3. New York, Harper & Row, 1971, p. 399.
97. Werner, S. C.: The severe eye changes of Graves' disease. J.A.M.A. 177:551–555 (Aug. 7) 1961.
98. Werner, S. C.: Prednisone in emergency treatment of malignant exophthalmos. Lancet 1:1004–1007 (May 7) 1966.
99. Werner, S. C. (Moderator): Two panel discussions on hyperthyroidism. I. Hyperthyroidism in the pregnant woman and the neonate. J. Clin. Endocr. 27:1637–1654 (Nov.) 1967.
100. Werner, S. C. (Moderator): Two panel discussions on hyperthyroidism. II. Etiology and treatment of hyperthyroidism in the adult. J. Clin. Endocr. 27:1763–1777 (Dec.) 1967.
101. Werner, S. C.: Classification of the eye changes of Graves' disease. J. Clin. Endocr. 29:982–984 (July) 1969.
102. Werner, S. C., Hamilton, H., and Nemeth, M.: Graves' disease: Hyperthyroidism or hyperpituitarism? J. Clin. Endocr. 12:1561–1571 (Dec.) 1952.
103. Werner, S. C., and Ingbar, S. H. (eds.): The Thyroid. Ed. 3. New York, Harper & Row, 1971, p. 505.
104. Werner, S. C., and Ingbar, S. H. (eds.): The Thyroid. Ed. 3. New York, Harper & Row, 1971, p. 507.
105. Werner, S. C., Spooner, M., and Hamilton, H.: Further evidence that hyperthyroidism (Graves' disease) is not hyperpituitarism: Effects of triiodothyronine and sodium iodide. J. Clin. Endocr. 15:715–723 (June) 1955.
106. Wool, M. S.: The investigation and treatment of hyperthyroidism. Surg. Clin. N. Amer. 50:545–558 (June) 1970.
107. Zellmann, H. E.: Malignant exophthalmos. Med. Clin. N. Amer. 53:469–477 (March) 1969.
108. Zellmann, H. E., and Sedgwick, C. E.: Hashimoto's thyroiditis and Graves' disease. Coincidental occurrence. Lahey Clin. Found. Bull. 15:53–58, 1966.

Chapter Eight

NONTOXIC NODULAR GOITER (ADENOMATOUS GOITER)

Cornelius E. Sedgwick, M.D.

ETIOLOGY

From the pathologists' and surgeons' points of view relative to diagnosis and treatment, nontoxic nodular goiter is considered a single entity. In text[10] and literature it is usually divided into two types referable to geography and possible etiology. The commonest type is the endemic, nontoxic, iodine-deficient goiter most prevalent in mountainous areas where persons lack iodine in the diet. The second most common type is the sporadic goiter, usually but not always occurring outside the goiter belt, with no evidence of iodine deficiency; it may be the result of one or more causes not yet fully explained.

Although the pathogenesis of nodular formation is not clear, the concept originally described by Marine and Lenhart[3] is applicable to both types. Stimulated by repeated episodes of thyroid hormone deficiency, cycles of hyperplasia followed by involution produce the nodules.

Although the basic cause of nodular goiter is lack of iodine, many substances known as goitrogens have been incriminated as secondary factors influencing the severity of the disease process. Abnormal intake of fluorine may displace iodine for metabolism and produce endemic goiter.[11] Increased calcium in drinking water has been reported as a possible goitrogen by Taylor.[8,9] McCarrison[4,5] noted increased goiters in patients drinking water polluted with *Escherichia coli*. Drugs, particularly the antithyroid drugs, pyocyanate, perchlorate, and sulfonamide,[7] are known goitrogens. Although certain foods[1]—cabbage, turnips, and soybeans—may produce goiter in animals, they have not been proved to be goitrogens in man. Other explanations of the etiology of nontoxic nodular goiter are related to thyroid hormone production, that is, faulty iodine utilization or some other defect in hormone genesis.

CLINICAL ASPECTS

Nontoxic nodular goiter is more prevalent in women and may first become apparent at the time of puberty. The signs and symptoms of nodular goiter are related to its size and location. Small nodular goiter, particularly in obese women, may go unnoticed. Larger goiters may be unsightly and become a cosmetic problem. Low lying goiters may enlarge, grow into the mediastinum, and, by pressure, cause deviation of the trachea and respiratory embarrassment. The correct clinical diagnosis of nodular goiter is related to the skill and experience of the clinician. I have found the most effectual method of palpating the thyroid to be that described by Lahey and Hare[2] (Fig. 8–1): The physician faces the seated patient. With the thumb of the right hand exerting pressure on the lateral margin of the thyroid cartilage on the opposite side of the

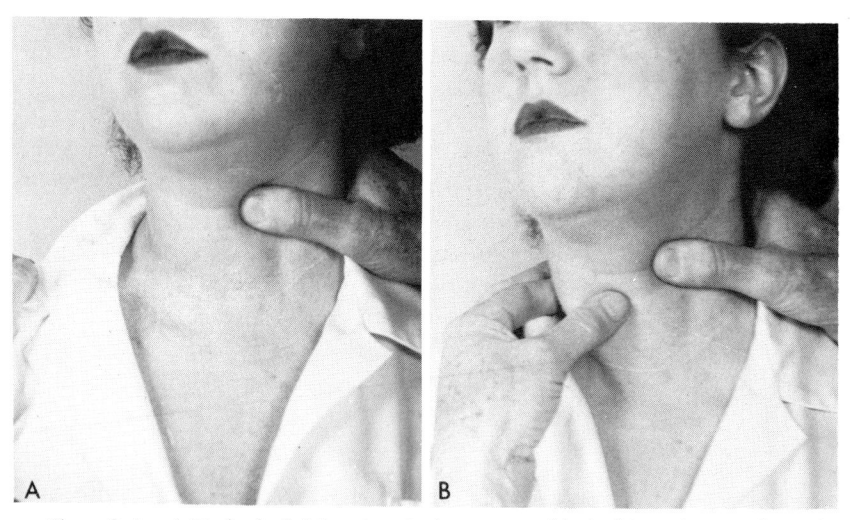

Figure 8–1. *A*, Method of dislocating the larynx out of its bed in order to palpate the lobe of the thyroid through and through. The finger pressing the larynx out of its position is applied against the thyroid cartilage where it will not produce coughing or choking. Note how definitely the right thyroid lobe can be dislocated outward for through-and-through palpation.

B, Method of palpating the dislocated right lobe. Note the index finger behind the right sternocleidomastoid muscle, relaxed by turning the chin to the right. The examining thumb is applied over the thyroid lobe in front as the larynx is dislocated to the right by the thumb of the other hand. When the patient is asked to swallow, the thyroid lobe to be palpated ascends and descends between the index finger and the thumb so that it can be thoroughly palpated for a nodule, the consistency that goes with hyperplasia characteristic of hyperthyroidism or the ligneous type of infiltration characteristic of thyroiditis. (From Lahey, F. H., and Hare, H. F.: J.A.M.A. *145*:696–697, 1951.)

NONTOXIC NODULAR GOITER

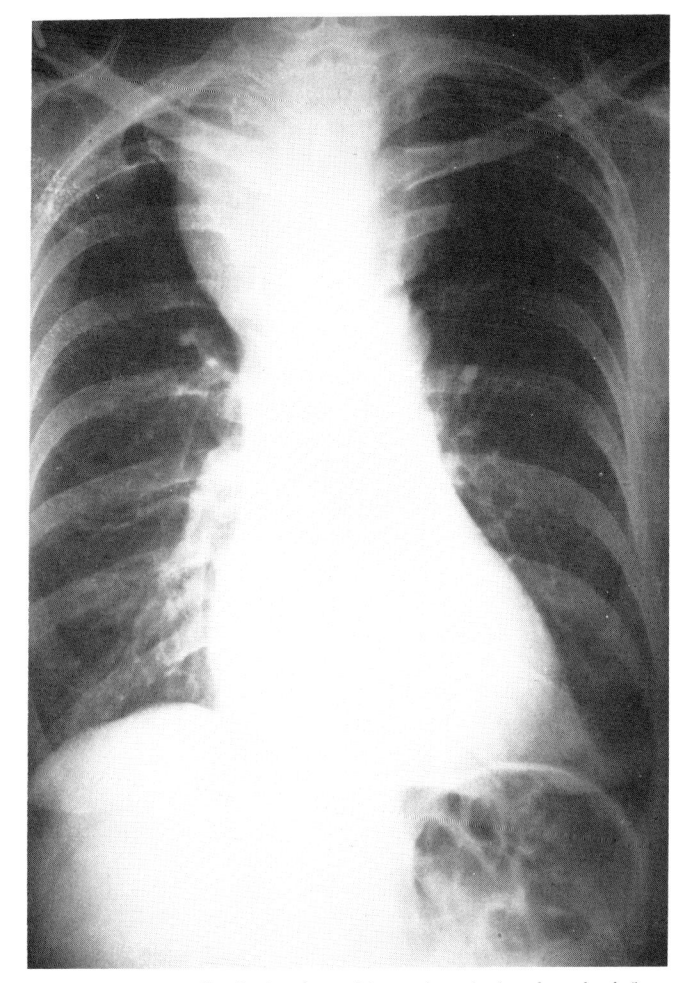

Figure 8-2. Mediastinal goiter with trachea deviated to the left.

lobe to be examined, he dislocates the larynx from its bed. When the patient swallows, the thyroid lobe ascends and descends between the left index finger and thumb of the examiner. The size, presence of nodules, and consistency of the thyroid are then determined.

DIAGNOSTIC AIDS

Further information relative to the nodular goiter is obtained by diagnostic x-ray study and scintiscan with radioactive iodine. A roentgenogram of the neck, chest, and mediastinum may reveal calcification in the region of the goiter. Deviation of the trachea or the presence of a mediastinal shadow suggests substernal goiter (Fig. 8-2). A scintiscan with ^{131}I of the neck and mediastinum may confirm the presence of goiter. (See Chapter Six.)

DIFFERENTIAL DIAGNOSIS

Nodularity of the thyroid may suggest nontoxic nodular goiter, chronic thyroiditis, adenoma, or malignant disease. The burden of proof rests on the clinician to rule out malignancy. The only sure method of diagnosis is tissue biopsy. In clinical material the reported incidence of carcinoma in nodular goiter varies from less than 1 percent to 17 percent, depending upon the selection of cases. Postmortem examination of unselected cases yields an incidence of 1.79 percent.[6] Obviously all nontoxic nodular goiters, particularly small asymptomatic goiters, should not be removed merely to establish a tissue diagnosis. Needle aspiration biopsy is reserved for those clinicians and pathologists adept at this diagnostic procedure. Malignant degeneration in nontoxic nodular goiters should be suspected if only a single nodule is palpated (especially in the young female), if a particular nodule is hard (the presence of calcium does not rule out malignant disease), and if the nodule is associated with rapid growth, pressure, hoarseness, pain, or tenderness. (The reader is referred to the chapters on chronic thyroiditis and thyroid tumors.)

TREATMENT

The treatment of nontoxic nodular goiter may be iodine given orally, thyroid extract for suppression, or surgical removal. Although increased oral intake of iodine is effectual prophylaxis for endemic nodular goiter, it is disappointing in producing regression, particularly in longstanding, large, nodular goiters. Regression from the use of thyroid extracts likewise is disappointing in most cases; it is most effective in young patients with nonfunctioning nodules. It must be emphasized that well differentiated carcinoma also responds to suppression and may be masked by thyroid extract therapy in its early stages when surgical removal is most effective. The surgical indications in nontoxic nodular goiter are for cosmetic reasons, suspicion of cancer, production of respiratory symptoms, and substernal goiters showing evidence of tracheal deviation and growth.

REFERENCES

1. Fertman, M. B., and Curtis, G. M.: Foods and the genesis of goiter. J. Clin. Endocr. 11:1361–1382 (Nov.) 1951.
2. Lahey, F. H., and Hare, H. F.: Malignancy in adenomas of thyroid. J.A.M.A. 145:689–695 (March 10) 1951.

3. Marine, D., and Lenhart, C. H.: Observations and experiments on the so-called thyroid carcinoma of brook trout (Salvelinus fontinalis) and its relation to ordinary goitre. J. Exp. Med. 12:311–327 (May 1) 1910.
4. McCarrison, R.: Observations on endemic goitre in the Chitral and Gilgit Valleys. Lancet 1:1110–1111 (April 21) 1906.
5. McCarrison, R.: Further researches on the etiology of endemic goitre. Quart. J. Med. 2:279–287 (April) 1908.
6. Silverberg, S. G., and Vidone, R. A.: Carcinoma of the thyroid in surgical and postmortem material. Analysis of 300 cases at autopsy and literature review. Ann. Surg. 164:291–299 (Aug.) 1966.
7. Stanbury, J. B., and Wyngaarden, J. B.: Effect of perchlorate on the human thyroid gland. Metabolism 1:533–539 (Nov.) 1952.
8. Taylor, S.: Calcium as a goitrogen. J. Clin. Endocr. 14:1412–1442 (Nov.) 1954.
9. Taylor, S.: Genesis of the thyroid nodule. Brit. Med. Bull. 16:102–105 (May) 1960.
10. Werner, S. C., and Ingbar, S. H. (eds.): The Thyroid, A Fundamental and Clinical Text. 3rd ed. New York, Harper & Row, 1971.
11. Wilson, D. C.: Fluorine in the aetiology of endemic goitre. Lancet 1:211–212 (Feb. 15) 1941.

Chapter Nine

THYROIDITIS

Bentley P. Colcock, M.D.

Many patients with chronic thyroiditis require some form of surgery. They may require a thyroidectomy to remove a prominent goiter; others can be relieved of annoying pressure symptoms in the neck only by an operative procedure. Many of these patients have a localized hard mass in the thyroid gland. Only histological examination of an adequate amount of tissue from this particular area will definitely rule out carcinoma.

CLASSIFICATION

Thyroiditis has been classified into five types: (1) acute suppurative thyroiditis, (2) subacute thyroiditis (acute thyroiditis, de Quervain's thyroiditis, or granulomatous thyroiditis), (3) Hashimoto's thyroiditis or struma lymphomatosa, (4) Riedel's thyroiditis, and (5) nonspecific thyroiditis. In many patients this inflammatory (or inflammatory-like) condition is not easy to classify. Some pathologists would place all patients with thyroiditis in one or another of the first four categories. Our pathologists prefer to classify the lesion as nonspecific chronic thyroiditis when it meets the strict criteria laid down by Hashimoto. Thus, figures regarding the incidence of Hashimoto's, Riedel's, or nonspecific thyroiditis vary a great deal. Many patients are not typical of any one type. Fortunately for surgeons, this confusion regarding precise classification does not greatly affect the surgical management of these patients.

Acute Suppurative Thyroiditis

Very rarely an acute suppurative process in the neck leads to an abscess in the thyroid gland. The abscess should, of course, be incised and drained. Care must be taken, however, not to mistake the fever associated with pain and tenderness of the gland so often seen in subacute thyroiditis as indicating an abscess. Patients with subacute thyroiditis (de Quervain's disease) seldom require operation even though they may be slow in responding to medical treatment. Only if definite fluctuation can be felt should incision and drainage of the thyroid gland be considered. Even then, it would be wise to prove the presence of pus by aspiration with a needle.

Subacute Thyroiditis

Means et al.[7] have defined subacute thyroiditis as "a self-limited inflammatory condition of the thyroid which may last for a week or two, or for several months. It has a marked tendency to recur. There is an associated depression of normal iodine metabolism in the involved gland." The etiology is obscure. The fact that it may follow an upper respiratory tract infection or a sore throat suggests a viral origin or an allergic reaction precipitated by the infection. They point out that the disease has occurred in epidemic form during an epidemic of mumps. Numerous attempts to culture viruses from patients whose disease was not associated with mumps have failed. This type of thyroiditis is not common. It is usually easy to diagnose, and the treatment is conservative; heat, rest, and aspirin or codeine will relieve the patient. Desiccated thyroid is given to patients who continue to have a tender, large thyroid gland. If these measures fail, the fever and malaise continue, and the gland remains enlarged and tender, prednisone may be effective. Prednisone (or its equivalent), 10 to 20 mg., is given each day for one week; then the dosage is reduced slowly during the next month.

The only indication for operation would be the occasional patient in whom it is impossible to exclude carcinoma. An example is the patient who has few if any symptoms, but who has a hard, localized mass in one lobe of the thyroid gland. A conservative subtotal lobectomy removing the involved area will definitely rule out cancer.

Chronic Thyroiditis

It is in patients with chronic thyroiditis, whether Hashimoto's, Riedel's, or nonspecific, that the need for operation most often occurs. It should be kept in mind that the pathologist may have difficulty in classifying the patient's disease even after he has studied the tissue. The following varieties of chronic thyroiditis are well known. They, plus the many cases that fall in between, account for the varied clinical picture and operative findings.

Hashimoto's Struma. In 1912 Hashimoto reported four cases of a new type of goiter that he called struma lymphomatosa. In recent years many papers have appeared indicating that this type of chronic thyroiditis is an auto-immune disease. However, as Bell[1] has stated, the cause is still uncertain. Immune mechanisms have been recognized, but their role in pathogenesis remains unsettled. Abnormalities found in serum protein and flocculation tests are probably secondary manifestations of the immune process. For treatment he recommends the long-term administration of daily doses of desiccated thyroid (120 to 140 mg.) and the avoidance of large amounts of iodide. Iodides aggravate an already existing defective organification of trapped iodide. This internist with long experience in the treatment of thyroid disease points out that surgical excision is indicated when carcinoma cannot be excluded or when thyroid extract fails to relieve pressure symptoms or cause shrinkage of a large goiter.

Priebe and Patterson[9] emphasize that Hashimoto's struma is not a rare form of thyroid disease. Our experience would confirm this if many of our cases classified as nonspecific thyroiditis were included. During a 20-year period (1945 through 1964) 975 patients were seen at the Lahey Clinic because of thyroiditis. Operations were performed on 70 percent. Most of the patients who were operated on had Hashimoto's or nonspecific chronic thyroiditis.

Almost all patients with chronic thyroiditis are women. In our series, 92 percent were women, and the majority were in the fourth and fifth decades of life. The age distribution ranged from 8 to 82 years. In 54 percent the chief complaint was a diffusely enlarged or a nodular thyroid gland.

In the typical patient with Hashimoto's thyroiditis, the gland is not so hard as it is in carcinoma, nonspecific, or Riedel's thyroiditis. It usually has a firm, rubbery consistency. At operation the gland may have the appearance as well as the feel of liver tissue. In making the diagnosis, it is helpful if the symmetry of the gland is preserved. The superior poles, inferior poles, both lobes, and isthmus are enlarged but have the shape of a normal thyroid gland.

Unfortunately many patients with chronic thyroiditis do not present this classic textbook picture. In 85 percent of our 975 patients, the gland was found to be enlarged, and in 83 percent it was described as hard. In 52 percent it was definitely nodular. In two thirds of Priebe's and Patterson's[9] patients, the enlargement was diffuse, and in one third it was localized. Symptoms of hypothyroidism were present in 4.2 percent. Symptoms of hyperthyroidism were occasionally present in patients with subacute thyroiditis, but were rarely seen in patients with chronic thyroiditis. Although clinical hypothyroidism is not common, laboratory tests may indicate that thyroid function is on the low side. Many patients complain of pressure in the neck. Blake and Sturgeon[2] reported 75 percent of their patients had symptoms such as dyspnea, choking, cough, dysphasia, or a husky voice.

Riedel's Struma. Patients with typical Riedel's struma are uncommon. They have a hard, nodular, more or less fixed goiter. Pressure symptoms are common, and these patients are likely to be somewhat older than those with Hashimoto's or nonspecific thyroiditis.

Nonspecific Thyroiditis. Our pathologists believe that any patient in whom the histological picture does not fit the original description by

Hashimoto or Riedel should be given a diagnosis of nonspecific thyroiditis. This explains why so many of our patients with chronic thyroiditis fall in this category.

DIAGNOSIS

A diagnosis of chronic thyroiditis can often be made on the physical examination of the thyroid gland. If the patient is a woman and the gland (though enlarged) is symmetrical and of uniform firmness or hardness throughout, the patient almost certainly has thyroiditis. A careful follow-up will establish the diagnosis. Thyroid extract may cause the goiter to shrink; it may relieve pressure symptoms in the neck. If the patient is asymptomatic and the goiter is not large (or shrinks sufficiently with therapy), no surgery is indicated. A needle biopsy may be performed if desired, but the risk of carcinoma is small. This is not true, however, when the thyroid gland is hard, irregular, or nodular.

INDICATIONS FOR SURGERY

Removal of a Goiter

When the gland is large and fails to shrink with desiccated thyroid extract, thyroidectomy may well be justified for cosmetic reasons alone. Today, thyroidectomy carries a negligible risk and is associated with few serious complications. Most of these patients are women, and their neck is always exposed to view. Even a moderate-sized goiter is likely to be of concern to the patient, her family, and her friends.

Persistence of Pressure Symptoms in the Neck

Thyroid extract may fail to relieve the annoying sense of constriction (or other "pressure symptoms") in the neck. This will be true for almost all patients with Riedel's struma and for many patients with nonspecific thyroiditis or Hashimoto's struma. When these symptoms persist, a subtotal thyroidectomy, or at least removal of the isthmus, is indicated.

To Rule Out Carcinoma

As pointed out previously, the gland may be only slightly enlarged in patients with chronic thyroiditis. It is often diffusely involved, and nodules or discrete masses are not palpable. The likelihood of carcinoma being present in these patients is small. If they are carefully followed up, it is *not* likely that the tragic mistake of failing to diagnose a cancer of the thyroid will be made. However, in patients who have an asymmetrical gland or in whom one area or lobe is larger and harder than the rest of the gland, only a biopsy will rule out cancer.

A few surgeons have advocated the use of the Silverman (or similar type) needle for biopsy. Crile and Hazard[3] followed up 222 patients with Hashimoto's struma and stated: "No micro carcinoma theoretically present in any of these patients developed into clinical malignancy." (All received 2 to 3 grains of desiccated thyroid daily.) In our experience, carcinoma was present in 1.7 percent of the 975 patients and occurred only in patients with nonspecific chronic thyroiditis. No thyroid carcinoma was found in patients with Hashimoto's struma. We would agree, therefore, that "struma lymphomatosa (Hashimoto's disease) treated by thyroid hormones should not be regarded as a premalignant lesion." We do not agree, however, that surgery is rarely indicated in patients with Hashimoto's struma (or nonspecific thyroiditis) or that "needle biopsy is a safe and effective way of ruling out malignancy." Carcinoma of the thyroid is frequently surrounded by tissue with histological characteristics of thyroiditis. It is difficult to be certain that the needle has penetrated beyond this surrounding tissue into the area under suspicion. Although the number of patients in whom we have employed needle biopsy is small, this has happened in our experience. Only because we are highly suspicious of thyroid cancer in a hard nodular goiter has serious error been prevented.

Woolner, McConahey and Beahrs[11] have also recommended the use of needle biopsy to rule out carcinoma. However, it should be noted that they believe all patients with Riedel's struma should have an exploratory operation. They also operated upon one third of their patients with Hashimoto's struma. They found 18 instances of papillary carcinoma in 605 patients with Hashimoto's struma. In 11 it was occult, and only two patients had metastases to adjacent lymph nodes. They concluded that since papillary carcinoma, especially if occult, is curable by surgical procedures, the lives of these patients were not endangered by "predominantly medical" treatment. From their own experience, a better conclusion would have been "a careful choice of medical treatment."

The risk of misdiagnosing cancer of the thyroid as chronic thyroiditis is a very real one. Hendrick[5] reported five patients in whom a carcinoma of the thyroid was overlooked by a needle biopsy. Carcinoma was also found in three other patients who had been diagnosed elsewhere as having Hashimoto's struma. Lindsey and Dailey,[4, 6] Pollock and Sprong,[8] and Schlicke et al.[10] have emphasized the fallibility of needle biopsy in ruling out carcinoma in these patients. Both carcinoma and thyroiditis occur largely in women. In Schlicke's study, one of four patients in each group had pressure symptoms, and a comparable number had symptoms suggesting hyperthyroidism not supported by thyroid function tests. Pollock and Sprong[8] found associated malignant disease in 11 percent of 52 patients with Hashimoto's struma. Schlicke et al.[10] found nine instances of carcinoma in 103 patients with Hashimoto's struma.

There is another factor that often arises in connection with needle biopsy. Many pathologists—even those experienced in thyroid pathology—may not be able to rule out carcinoma based on what they see in the small amount of tissue obtained by a needle. The important point is not whether the incidence of cancer in chronic thyroiditis is 1.7 percent, 9 percent, 11 percent, or somewhere in between: it is, does the patient in whom you find a hard mass in the thyroid gland have chronic thyroiditis *or* carcinoma? We must also keep in mind that whatever the effect of desiccated thyroid is on occult microscopic carcinoma, it does not cure clinical cancer of the thyroid. Even if the tumor is a papillary adenocarcinoma, if it is not removed it will eventually invade the trachea and the esophagus and become incurable. It may take 15 years to do so.

OPERATIVE PROCEDURE

For most patients a conservative subtotal thyroidectomy is the procedure of choice. It removes an objectionable goiter, relieves pressure symptoms in the neck, and provides ample tissue to establish the diagnosis. Priebe and Patterson[9] found four patients with recurrences after removal of the isthmus or one lobe and concluded that the resection should remove more than 50 percent but less than 75 percent of the gland. Lahey pointed out many years ago that suture of the medial border of the sternothyroid muscles to the lateral border of the trachea on each side would help to prevent the regeneration of thyroid tissue across the trachea. The surgeon should keep in mind that in many patients with chronic thyroiditis, the recurrent nerves are likely to be adherent to the posterior surface of the gland. Forceful retraction of the thyroid lobe during its subtotal removal may cause a temporary or even a permanent vocal cord paralysis on that side. For this reason we do not approximate the thyroid remnant to the lateral border of the trachea as we do when operating on patients with Graves' disease. Since bleeding is rarely a problem and the remaining thyroid tissue is underactive, I also omit ligation of the inferior thyroid arteries. All patients with chronic thyroiditis are given desiccated thyroid extract after operation. A careful follow-up will determine the daily dose required.

SUMMARY

In many patients with chronic thyroiditis, a hard, irregular, or nodular goiter develops. Such a goiter is the first and often the only sign of cancer of the thyroid. The differential diagnosis must be made by histological examination of an adequate amount of tissue from the suspicious area. A conservative subtotal thyroidectomy is the most certain means of ruling out carcinoma. It is also the best treatment for a patient with chronic thyroiditis who continues to have an unsightly goiter, or pressure symptoms in the neck, despite the administration of thyroid extract.

REFERENCES

1. Bell, G. O.: Hashimoto's thyroiditis (struma lymphomatosa). Surg. Clin. N. Amer. 42:647-653 (June) 1962.
2. Blake, K. W., and Sturgeon, C. T.: Struma lymphomatosa. Surg. Gynec. Obstet. 97:312-317 (Sept.) 1953.
3. Crile, G., Jr., and Hazard, J. B.: Incidence of cancer in struma lymphomatosa. Surg. Gynec. Obstet. 115:101-103 (July) 1962.
4. Dailey, M. E., Lindsay, S., and Skahen, R.: The relation of thyroid neoplasms to Hashimoto's disease of the thyroid gland. Arch. Surg. 70:291-297 (Feb.) 1955.
5. Hendrick, J. W.: Diagnosis and treatment of thyroiditis. Ann. Surg. 144:176-187 (Aug.) 1956.
6. Lindsay, S., Dailey, M. E., Friedlander, J., et al.: Chronic thyroiditis: Clinical and pathologic study of 354 patients. J. Clin. Endocr. 12:1578-1600 (Dec) 1952.
7. Means, J. H., DeGroot, L. J., and Stanbury, J. B.: The Thyroid and Its Diseases. 3rd ed. New York, McGraw-Hill Book Company, 1963, pp. 420-461.
8. Pollock, W. F., and Sprong, D. H., Jr.: The rationale of thyroidectomy for Hashimoto's thyroiditis, a premalignant lesion. West. J. Surg. 66:17-20 (Jan.-Feb.) 1958.
9. Priebe, C. J., Jr., and Patterson, H. A.: Surgical aspects of chronic thyroiditis. Ann. Surg. 150:965-975 (Dec.) 1959.
10. Schlicke, C. P., Hill, J. E., and Schultz, G. F.: Carcinoma in chronic thyroiditis. Surg. Gynec. Obstet. 111:552-556 (Nov.) 1960.
11. Woolner, L. B., McConahey, W. M., and Beahrs, O. H.: Struma lymphomatosa (Hashimoto's thyroiditis) and related thyroidal disorders. J. Clin. Endocr. 19:53-83 (Jan.) 1959.

Chapter Ten

THYROID TUMORS

Cornelius E. Sedgwick, M.D.
and
John R. Bookwalter, M.D.

The management of thyroid tumors by the surgeon demands close consultation with a pathologist who is experienced and competent in thyroid disease. Often the appearance of excised abnormal thyroid tissue is deceiving. A papillary or follicular carcinoma or adenoma appearing as a well circumscribed nodule may be difficult to distinguish from a nodular or endemic goiter. As in few other malignancies, the surgeon must select the indicated procedure based on the interpretation of the frozen section by the pathologist. Furthermore, the prognosis, to a great extent, depends upon the pathologic classification of the tumor. A detailed discussion of thyroid tumor pathology is found in Chapter Four.

CLINICAL EVALUATION OF THE PATIENT WITH A THYROID NODULE

Patients presenting with a thyroid nodule may be conveniently divided into two groups: The first group consists of patients who have symptoms related to the nodule; the second group has asymptomatic nodules discovered merely by their appearance or unexpectedly by routine physical examination. The symptomatic nodules occur more often in patients with the more diffuse type of thyroid disease, such as hyperthyroidism, multinodular goiter, acute and chronic thyroiditis, medullary thyroid cancer, and more extensive neoplasms. The second group, the relatively asymptomatic patients, will present with well circumscribed lesions suggesting benign and malignant neoplasm. Thus, the discovery of an asymptomatic mass in the thyroid, either by the patient or by a physician, carries a distinct possibility of neoplasm and puts the burden of correct diagnosis on the consultant. A careful history is imperative in the differential diagnosis of neoplasm from other forms of thyroid disease. Important questions to be answered are: How was the nodule first discovered? How was it treated? Is the enlargement associated with symptoms of hypothyroidism or hyperthyroidism? Is there pain or discomfort in the neck? Is there hoarseness or difficulty in swallowing? Has the patient ever received radiation to the neck? Is there a history of other endocrine abnormalities? Is the nodule enlarging?

Change in size of a thyroid nodule has important diagnostic value. Many malignant tumors may show very little change in size for years, and then suddenly, without obvious cause, begin to grow. The solitary, painless nodule that has been present for sometime, but which has recently increased in size, is almost always neoplastic, with the risk of malignancy increasing with age, especially after menopause.

A history of preexisting known thyroid disease is important. It is interesting that many patients with follicular adenocarcinoma have a history of preexisting thyroid disease many years before the diagnosis was established. The duration of thyroid enlargement before operation, however, does not assist in deciding whether cervical lymph nodes contain metastatic disease. Occasionally a patient who has been given thyroid extract for suppression of an adenomatous goiter discontinues the medication for some reason and sometime later presents with a history of recent growth after a long period of quiescence. Usually this occurs within a few months to a year after cessation of the medication.

A history of radiation therapy to the neck either for inflammatory disease of the thyroid or thymus enlargement in the newborn is associated with a higher incidence of thyroid malignancy in children and young adults.[17, 31]

Subjective symptoms of abnormal thyroid function are not usually associated with neoplasms of the thyroid. A history of nervousness, weight loss, heat intolerance, easy fatigability, and onset of a fine tremor may be associated with Graves' disease, toxic nodular goiter, or hyperfunctioning adenoma. Conversely, cold sensitivity, slow speech with hoarse voice, and excessive menstruation may be the result of hypothyroidism secondary to chronic thyroiditis. It should be emphasized, however, that the presence of hyperthyroidism or hypothyroidism does not rule out the presence of malignant disease, since we have seen cancer of the thyroid in patients with myxedema as well as in patients with Graves' disease.

Pain is of diagnostic importance in evaluating a thyroid nodule. With the exception of medullary carcinoma, thyroid neoplasms are rarely painful. Pain associated with the sudden appearance of a mass in the thyroid is frequently indicative of hemorrhage into an adenoma with later cystic degeneration. Pain and tenderness of the entire gland is most often associated with acute or subacute thyroiditis, but medullary carcinoma can also present with diffuse low grade pain and tenderness.

Hoarseness is a significant sign, often indicating invasion of the recurrent nerve by tumor. Such patients must be examined by direct or mirror laryngoscopy to rule out paralysis of the vocal cord. Patients with thyroid malignancy who have hoarseness secondary to tumor invasion of the recurrent laryngeal nerve have a very poor prognosis. Although this most often occurs in undifferentiated tumor, we have seen it in papillary carcinoma as well.

Difficulty in swallowing may be difficult to evaluate. Dysphagia is a late manifestation of thyroid malignancy and indicates actual fixation of the gland to the surrounding structures. Globus hystericus in a patient with a thyroid nodule or mass may make it difficult to determine if the thyroid lesion is responsible for the dysphagia. Usually thyroid lesions causing dysphagia are either quite large or obviously fixed to underlying tissue. In the latter case, thyroid malignancy is almost certain.

A history of other endocrine disorders in a patient presenting with a thyroid nodule or with diffuse tenderness should alert one to the possibility of medullary carcinoma of the thyroid, since a significant percentage of these patients have associated endocrine disorders, most commonly pheochromocytoma (often familial and bilateral), hyperparathyroidism, Cushing's disease, carcinoid, and diabetes.

PHYSICAL EXAMINATION

The physical examination of the patient with a thyroid nodule is critical. It permits the nodule to be classified in several ways that will affect the manner in which the patient is treated. The recommended technique for examining a thyroid gland is described in Chapter Three under "Nodular Goiter." The size, consistency, degree of tenderness, and location of the nodule are determined as the patient swallows. Careful assessment must be made to ascertain whether one is dealing with a true solitary nodule or a multinodular goiter, since this distinction determines whether surgery is advised or further observation is recommended. Careful search for enlarged cervical nodes is made. Frequently, particularly with differentiated carcinoma, cervical lymphadenopathy is more prominent than the primary thyroid mass. Finally, the patient should be examined for stigmata of hyperthyroidism and myxedema.

OTHER DIAGNOSTIC AIDS

A roentgenogram of the chest will often demonstrate substernal extension of the goiter, deviation and narrowing of the trachea, or metastatic lesions in the lung.

An accurate index of thyroid function should be obtained to determine the current metabolic level and to provide a baseline for further studies. Formerly the basal metabolism test was used extensively at the Lahey Clinic. With all its difficulties, this test had the one advantage of being insensitive to the various iodine compounds used so frequently in modern diagnostic radiology (Chapter Five). At present we are using the serum thyroxine (T4) test because it, too, is not affected by exogenous iodine compounds. In addition, a protein-bound iodine test is of value in determining thyroid function as well as determining the validity of radioiodine uptake and scans. The difference in the results obtained from the protein-bound iodine test and the serum thyroxine test determinations may indicate that the level of exogenous iodine is too great to permit a satisfactory thyroid scan at a given time. Finally, at an appropriate time the thyroid scan should be performed to determine the level of activity of the nodule and to check for the presence of other nodules that may, clinically, have gone undetected on physical examination.[1] The great advantage of the thyroid scan is that it is an objective and reproducible method of following the course of thyroid disease and the response to treatment. For maximum benefit it must be correlated closely with the physical examination. It should be realized that the smallest nodule that will show up on a scan is about 1.0 to 1.5 cm., depending on location within the gland. Thus, a small cold nodule, which carries a higher risk of malignancy, may appear as normal or with minimal hypofunction on scan. Thyroid scanning is discussed in detail in Chapter Six.

MANAGEMENT

Our plan of management of thyroid neoplasm is based on the pathological classification of the tumor or the degree of malignancy, the clinical classification of the tumor or the degree of invasion (Table 10-1), the age of the patient,[5] and the location of the tumor within the thyroid gland. Treatment for each patient must be individualized (Table 10-2).

The histological or pathological classification of malignant tumors grades the degree of malignancy, with papillary adenocarcinoma being the least malignant, follicular adenocarcinoma next, medullary carcinoma more so, and the undifferentiated carcinoma the most malignant (Table 10-3). The papillary adenocarcinomas are further subdivided into adenomas with minimal capsular, lymphatic, or blood vessel invasion which show a lesser degree of malignancy. The clinical stage grades the extent of the tumor both clinically and at the time of surgery, that is, is the tumor confined to the thyroid gland, the lymphatics, or has it involved surrounding neck structures or metastasized outside the neck? In selecting the appropriate operative procedure, the surgeon

Table 10-1. Clinical Stages of Thyroid Cancer

Stage I.	Tumor confined to the thyroid gland.
Stage II.	Tumor confined to the thyroid gland and regional lymph nodes.
Stage III.	Tumor invades the deep structures of the neck with or without nodal metastases.
Stage IV.	Any of the above with distant metastases.

Table 10–2. Management of Thyroid Cancer

STAGE	DIFFERENTIATED THYROID CANCER	MEDULLARY THYROID CANCER	UNDIFFERENTIATED THYROID CANCER
I	1. Radical subtotal lobectomy on any lobe grossly involved with tumor 2. Subtotal lobectomy on contralateral lobe without gross tumor 3. Lifetime thyroid suppression	1. Radical subtotal lobectomy on any lobe grossly involved with tumor 2. Subtotal lobectomy on contralateral lobe without gross tumor 3. Lifetime thyroid suppression 4. Consider prophylactic node dissection	1. Radical subtotal lobectomy on any lobe grossly involved with tumor 2. Subtotal lobectomy on contralateral lobe without gross tumor 3. Lifetime thyroid suppression 4. Consider prophylactic node dissection
II	1, 2, and 3 as for stage I 4. Node dissection in affected area (neck or mediastinum or both) 5. Consider ablation of thyroid remnant with radioactive iodine and treatment with radioactive iodine	1, 2, and 3 as for stage I 4. Node dissection in affected area (neck or mediastinum or both) 5. Consider megavoltage x-ray therapy	1, 2, and 3 as for stage I 4. Node dissection in affected area (neck or mediastinum or both) 5. Consider megavoltage x-ray therapy
III	1 and 2 as for stage I, removing as much gross tumor as possible 3. Lifetime thyroid suppression 4. Ablate thyroid remnant with radioactive iodine and use radioactive iodine as long as it is concentrated adequately 5. Use megavoltage radiotherapy to neck if residual tumor will not concentrate radioactive iodine	1 and 2 as for stage I, removing as much gross tumor as possible 3. Lifetime thyroid suppression 4. Use megavoltage x-ray therapy to neck	1. Biopsy only 2. Lifetime thyroid suppression 3. Use megavoltage x-ray therapy to neck
IV	1, 2, 3, and 4 as for stage III 5. Use megavoltage radiotherapy to metastatic lesions when radioactive iodine will not concentrate	1, 2, and 3 as for stage III 4. Use megavoltage x-ray therapy to metastatic lesions	1, 2, and 3 as for stage III 4. Use megavoltage x-ray therapy to metastatic lesions

Table 10-3. Thyroid Carcinoma in Order of Increasing Malignancy

---

Differentiated thyroid cancer
  Papillary carcinoma
  Mixed papillary and follicular carcinoma
  Follicular carcinoma

Medullary carcinoma

Undifferentiated thyroid carcinoma
  Small cell diffuse carcinoma
  Small cell compact carcinoma
  Large cell carcinoma

---

must know and appreciate the significance of the degree of malignancy (pathology classification) and the degree of invasion (clinical stage).

The tissue diagnosis for solitary nodule is obtained by a radical subtotal or near total lobectomy, with identification and protection of at least one parathyroid gland. A frozen section is obtained. If the lesion is benign or a low grade papillary adenocarcinoma, the operation is concluded. Some disagree with the concept that radical subtotal lobectomy is the best initial procedure for pathological examination. Others prefer excision of the nodule, believing that if it is benign, more extensive lobectomy is avoided. Still others prefer total lobectomy, believing that if it is malignant, it will not be necessary to perform further procedures on the lobe involved. This is particularly appropriate if facilities for examining a frozen section are not available and the surgeon must wait for permanent sections. We are not so overly concerned with the type of initial procedure as we are with obtaining the correct tissue diagnosis so that proper treatment can be instituted. If an adenoma with minimal capsular invasion is found, near total lobectomy will suffice. If the pathological classification is frank papillary or follicular adenocarcinoma with no evidence of involvement of lymphatics or adjacent structures, near total lobectomy on the involved side and a radical subtotal lobectomy on the opposite side may be performed.

Continuation of radical neck dissection in the absence of involvement of lymphatics is still a matter of controversy.[7, 9, 27] There are those who believe this is important because of reports that up to 30 percent of neck dissections performed with no evidence of involvement of lymphatics have been found to have lymph nodes invaded with tumor.[19] Others believe that radical neck dissection is indicated only when the adjacent cervical lymphatics are involved, and the stage of invasion is limited enough to permit resection of all tumor.[3] Total excision of all malignant tumor is frequently impossible because of invasion of the retropharyngeal or mediastinal nodes or massive widespread involvement of the cervical nodes. In such instances, radical neck dissection is abandoned, and all possible tumor is removed together with near total thyroidectomy on the side of the primary focus and radical subtotal thyroidectomy on the opposite side. Residual tumor may then be treated with radioactive iodine if it shows adequate uptake of the isotope or, if not, supervoltage x-ray therapy can be given.

Medullary carcinoma lies between the differentiated carcinomas and the undifferentiated carcinomas with respect to malignancy, and neck dissection should be combined with thyroidectomy in the presence of clinically suspicious neck nodes. Most of the undifferentiated carcinomas are beyond the limits of radical surgery. As much tumor as safely possible should be excised, and postoperative supervoltage x-ray therapy should be given. In some instances it is necessary to perform tracheostomy before radiation therapy because of the resulting tracheal edema in an already compromised airway.

The age of the patient must also be considered in selecting the appropriate operative procedure. Differentiated carcinoma of the same cell type in the adult seems to have a more malignant potential than it does in children.[5, 16, 27, 31] The 10-year survival rate of papillary carcinoma in children is considerably higher than that in adults. More aggressive surgery, therefore, is indicated relative to neck dissection in the adult. Individual node dissection, "berry picking," may be more appropriate in children. Finally, in deciding on the procedure to be performed, the location of the primary must be considered. A primary focus in the lower pole of a low lying goiter may show evidence of lymphatic involvement of the pretracheal lymph nodes draining into the mediastinum. A classic en bloc radical neck dissection would not remove these important lymphatics of the mediastinum. In such cases, mediastinal dissection should be combined with radical neck dissection if surgical removal of all tumor is possible.

We have five therapeutic modalities available to be used alone or more often in combination in treating carcinoma of the thyroid. They are surgery, radioactive iodine, supervoltage radiation, thyroid hormone, and chemotherapeutic agents. It must be stressed again that the use of these modalities is individualized for each patient, depending upon the pathological classification of the tumor, the stage of invasion, the age of the patient, and the location of the primary focus.

Surgical Excision

Surgery may consist of excision of the tumor, subtotal lobectomy, radical subtotal lobectomy, or near total lobectomy. Each must be defined. Excision means local excision of the adenoma or primary focus of about 70 percent of the lobe, leaving about 10 gm. of thyroid tissue and most of the posterior capsule from the superior to the inferior poles. Radical subtotal lobectomy is the removal of the tumor mass of 90 percent or more of the thyroid gland, leaving a small enough remnant and strip of posterior capsule to assure viability of at least one parathyroid gland. Near total lobectomy means removing all macroscopic thyroid tissue. What, to the surgeon, appears as a total lobectomy so often shows a minute particle of thyroid tissue on follow-up radioactive iodine scan that the term total thyroidectomy has been abandoned.

Our policy at the Lahey Clinic Foundation is to operate on practically all patients with solitary, painless, thyroid nodules after completing the work-up previously described, regardless of whether the scan reveals the lesion to take up the radioactive iodine more or less effectively than the surrounding tissue. We believe that although the probabilities of cancer are greater in men and in women under the age of 40 with cold nodules, the incidence of cancer is great enough in all groups to warrant surgical intervention. In some instances of multinodular goiter we administer suppressive therapy for a few months and postpone surgery if the lesion regresses, but we have found that this occurs in a disappointingly small percentage of patients. Surgical therapy resolves any doubt about the true nature of the lesion, and the mortality and morbidity are low enough to permit this approach with a very high degree of patient safety.

Those who disagree with this policy believe that the more common types of thyroid cancer, the papillary and follicular, grow slowly enough to permit a period of diagnostic evaluation of up to several months.[29] We agree for patients with suspected chronic thyroiditis with nodularity of diffusely nodular goiter, but the patient with a discrete nodule in an otherwise normal gland needs surgical exploration without the added expense and equivocation of a long and almost always unproductive diagnostic work-up. One of the frequently heard arguments against proceeding immediately with surgery is the feeling that the patient with a more differentiated type of thyroid cancer may die with the disease but not from it.[16, 32] Our mortality rate from disease for follicular carcinoma in patients followed for at least 10 years is about 25 percent, and for papillary carcinoma it is about 20 percent. These are good results when compared with most other types of malignancy, but the important fact is that these are the results in treated cases. We believe that despite the protracted course of the disease, the earlier the disease is recognized and treated as cancer the better the prognosis for the patient.[23, 28] Every attempt should be made to perform the proper surgical procedure before utilizing radioactive iodine or x-ray therapy in patients who have had previous thyroid surgery for either benign or malignant disease.

Selection of Operative Procedure

Near total thyroid lobectomy is our operation of choice for diagnostic purposes on all thyroid masses suspicious of malignancy. If the lesion is benign or small (less than 1 cm.) low grade papillary or follicular adenocarcinoma, no further surgery is performed. Usually, however, this is the first part of a more extensive surgical procedure. The goal of this procedure is to remove all tumor without compromising parathyroid function. The parathyroid glands are not spared on the side of the lesion if this cannot be done without compromising the removal of all cancer.

Contralateral Radical Subtotal Thyroid Lobectomy and Resection of the Isthmus. Contralateral radical subtotal thyroid lobectomy and resection of the isthmus is performed for all malignant lesions of the thyroid if feasible whether or not the opposite side and isthmus show tumor involvement. Studies have shown that the incidence of multicentric foci of malignancy in the contralateral lobe is as high as 80 to 90 percent.[22] Although it has been suggested that these foci of tumor do not necessarily have a growth potential, we believe that it adds little further risk or morbidity to excise the opposite lobe.

Neck Dissection. The status of neck dissection in the surgical therapy of thyroid cancer is uncertain at the present time, and the reasons will be discussed in the next section of this chapter. It is our current policy to perform neck dissection for known nodal metastases from differentiated thyroid cancers. The sternocleidomastoid muscle is spared if this can be done without compromising the completeness of the node dissection. Patients with metastases to both sides of the neck are treated with neck dissections performed a week or two apart. At the present time we are not performing prophylactic node dissections for differentiated thyroid tumors. In patients with medullary thyroid cancer we would proceed with neck dissection without a tissue diagnosis if there were any suspicion on clinical grounds of spread to the neck because of the high incidence of neck metastasis (over 50 percent) in patients with this tumor. In treating undifferentiated thyroid cancer, neck dissection is considered only if the primary form is small and well lateralized and there are no known distant metastases or macroscopic tumor left behind at the primary focus. There is little point in employing neck dissection in a patient with undifferentiated thyroid carcinoma unless the surgeon believes that all tumor can be removed and there is a good chance for cure.

Mediastinal Dissection. Because of the origin of the blood supply to the thyroid from the carotid arteries, it is rarely necessary to split the sternum to remove the thyroid gland itself, so that the use of the sternum-splitting incision to gain access to the mediastinum in patients with thyroid cancer is reserved primarily for removal of lymph node metastases. In patients with differentiated thyroid cancer or medullary cancer without distant metastases, mediastinal dissection is considered if the lesion is large, low lying, and centrally located. The presence of positive nodes in the neck, which are central and inferior to the gland, is an even stronger indication for mediastinal dissection. When undifferentiated thyroid cancer is found, mediastinal dissection is employed only when all tumor in the thyroid has been removed and the lesion is small, low lying, and centrally located. As with radical neck dissection, there is little reason to add mediastinal node dissection unless there is a good chance that the procedure will complete the removal of all tumor. The chapter on anatomy (Chapter Three) discusses more fully the lymphatic drainage of the thyroid as a rational basis for making decisions for employing neck or mediastinal dissections, or both, in the treatment of thyroid cancer.

Suppressive Therapy with Thyroid Extract

Suppressive therapy with thyroid extract is employed in all patients with cancer of the thyroid. With the advent of an increased understanding of the pituitary dependence of the thyroid gland in normal function, it was assumed that the more differentiated thyroid tumors were also thyroid-stimulating hormone-dependent to a certain extent. As a result of this assumption, most patients who have had a thyroid tumor excised are given thyroid extract or a suitable substitute for life following surgical therapy.[26] No controlled studies are available that clearly demonstrate the validity of this assumption, but it has nonetheless become one of the cornerstones of treatment of thyroid cancer. Currently our plan is to begin treating the patient on the second postoperative day with thyroid extract, 2 grains or its equivalent, and to increase the dose gradually, a grain at a time, until symptoms of hyperthyroidism develop. When this point is reached, the dose is reduced until the symptoms subside. The resultant daily dose becomes the maintenance dose for suppressive therapy. The reasons for the use of suppressive therapy are carefully explained to the patient to insure the permanent continuation of this regimen.

Radioactive Iodine

Radioactive iodine is used diagnostically to follow the activity of residual thyroid tissue following surgery for carcinoma of the thyroid and to treat metastatic lesions when such lesions, thought to be metastases, develop after surgery for well differentiated carcinoma of the thyroid. Thyroid hormone is stopped for several weeks, and the remaining normal thyroid tissue is ablated with about 30 to 80 mCi. radioactive iodine. After a period of one to three months, during which no thyroid replacement is given, another diagnostic scan is performed to see if the metastatic lesions will concentrate the isotope. In one well documented study, 30 percent of patients with well differentiated thyroid adenocarcinoma had metastases which concentrated radioactive iodine before thyroid ablation, 40 percent of patients concentrated radioactive iodine seven to nine weeks after ablation, and 13 percent did not concentrate radioactive iodine until three months after thyroid ablation.[20] The degree to which a metastatic lesion will concentrate radioactive iodine is important in how efficacious the therapy will be. In a patient who is given a 150 mCi. dose of radioactive iodine, a metastatic lesion that concentrates 0.1 percent of the dose per gram of tissue will receive 5,000 rads to the lesion, assuming a biologic half-life of four days for the radioactive iodine.[21] Thus, it is easily apparent why such therapy is chosen over conventional x-ray therapy when there is any chance of success.

In some cases thyroid-stimulating hormone is given for a day or two before radioactive iodine therapy to enhance further the uptake of radioactive iodine by the metastatic lesion. This is especially helpful in patients who cannot tolerate the usual period of abstinence from thyroid replacement before receiving radioactive iodine treatments. Radioactive iodine therapy is repeated at two- or three-month intervals until the metastatic lesion no longer concentrates the isotope. Concentration of the isotope by the lesions is followed by scintiscanning and by measuring the protein-bound iodine ^{131}I at periodic intervals after the dose is given as an indication of active uptake by functioning tumor tissue.

We believe strongly that it is worthwhile to consider radioactive iodine therapy in all instances of differentiated thyroid cancer when the presence of distant metastatic lesions (most commonly in the lungs) is suspected. Radioactive iodine has been of little or no benefit in the undifferentiated forms of thyroid cancer.

SUPERVOLTAGE EXTERNAL IRRADIATION

We recommend postoperative x-ray therapy to the neck with megavoltage irradiation in any patient with thyroid cancer in whom metastatic, invasive, or incompletely excised lesions are not amenable to further surgery or in whom radioactive iodine is not adequately concentrated. Despite the fact that this makes x-ray therapy our third line of defense in the treatment of thyroid cancer, it has been an extremely effective tool.[24] Many patients have obtained excellent long-term palliation and, in some instances, have been cured by external irradiation. Results are better, of course, with the more differentiated cancers, but we have a few well documented cases of incompletely excised undifferentiated tumors which responded dramatically to x-ray therapy; as a result, we offer it routinely to patients in whom surgery and radioactive iodine have proved inadequate. Less than one third of patients with undifferentiated tumors will respond for more than a few months, but radiation represents the last resort for this group of patients and is well worth trying.

Generally the dose varies between 4,000 and 6,000 rads given over four to six weeks.

Chemotherapy

Chemotherapy in the treatment of advanced metastatic or invasive thyroid cancer has been employed infrequently. However, a recent report by Gottlieb and Hill[12] suggests that chemotherapy may be of value for metastatic thyroid carcinoma. We can hope for considerable improvement in this area in the next decade as less toxic and more specific chemotherapeutic agents are developed.

Comment

In assessing the published results of the treatment of thyroid cancer,[14] it is well to keep in mind the criteria for an ideal study. The patient group should be as large as possible and clearly characterized as to age and sex. All patients should have a tissue diagnosis that, preferably, has recently been reviewed by one or two competent pathologists and brought into comformity with one of the currently accepted classification systems. The surgical procedures and other treatment modalities should be as uniform as possible so that conclusions based on their relative merits are valid. From a surgical point of view, this is best accomplished in studies in which the procedure was performed by or under the direction of the smallest possible number of surgeons. A precise definition of the surgical procedures performed should be included, a requirement that becomes increasingly important as larger numbers of surgeons become involved. The extent of the lesions at the time of surgery should be noted. The patient follow-up should be complete and should be carried on for the longest possible period of time. All patients in the series who die should have an autopsy to verify the presence and extent of disease.

The data involving the well differentiated thyroid cancers are probably best presented by comparison with life table data because of the high survival rates with these lesions, the low percentage of autopsies in most series, and the long period of time necessary to obtain a suitably large number of cases. When comparisons are made with life table data, the normal life expectancy curve can vary considerably, depending upon the ethnic, racial, and socioeconomic composition of the group. Ideally the normal life expectancy curve should be constructed for a group which is identical to the test group except for the presence of thyroid cancer. With the aid of a computer it has become possible to compose a normal life expectancy curve for a group which is matched exactly to the test group with respect to sex, age, and year of inclusion in the group (since life expectancy has increased dramatically in the last 40 years, this last factor has become important), so that the comparison of survival data by this technique becomes more valid as an accurate assessment of the mortality from the thyroid cancer alone. For the more malignant types of thyroid cancer, crude survival data are perfectly adequate to compare the results of the various treatment methods used at the present time because the mortality from the disease is so high that any treatment that represents a clear improvement will be singled out without too much difficulty.

DIFFERENTIATED THYROID CANCERS

This group of thyroid tumors is composed of papillary, follicular, and mixed papillary and follicular carcinomas and is the group in which the greatest degree of uncertainty exists concerning proper treatment. The principal reason for this is that the long-term survival rates are in the 70 to 90 percent range (Tables 10-4 and 10-5) as long as the primary focus of tumor is excised, so that extremely long and careful follow-up is necessary to document the success or failure of a given treatment plan. Because of the indolent nature of the disease and its relative rarity in the general population, treatment failures will not become evident for many years after the original surgical procedure. The rational evaluation of the relative merits of extensive versus limited resection, prophylactic node dissection, postoperative irradiation, and postoperative thyroid suppression has been hampered because of the necessarily longer periods required for adequate follow-up studies.

A second problem arising with differentiated thyroid cancers is that the diagnosis is often impossible to make on gross examination of the

Table 10-4. Representative Survival in Papillary Carcinoma of the Thyroid in Surgically Treated Cases

Study	Stage	10-Year Survival (%)	Number of Patients
Beahrs and Pasternak[2]	Occult or intrathyroid	Approx. 90	588
	Extrathyroid	Approx. 55	68
Buckwalter and Thomas[6]	All cases	Approx. 70	111
Frazell and Foote[11]	All cases	Approx. 69	106
Crile[10]	All cases	Approx. 85	74
Sutton et al.[25]	All cases	63	63
Hirabayashi and Lindsay[15]	All cases	84	250

Table 10-5. Survival in Follicular Carcinoma of the Thyroid in Surgically Treated Cases

Study	Stage	10-Year Survival (%)	Number of Patients
Beahrs and Pasternak[2]	Intrathyroidal	90	100
	Invasive	34	98
Buckwalter and Thomas[6]	All cases	Approx. 68	136
Sutton et al.[25]	All cases	34	48
Hirabayashi and Lindsay[15]	All cases	57	83

surgical specimen. In the Memorial series[11, 27] and in our own early experience before the use of the routine frozen section, as many as 50 percent of cases were not diagnosed as cancer until after operation, even though both surgical groups had had extensive experience with thyroid cancer. Thus, an unusually large responsibility for an intra-operative diagnosis is placed upon the pathologist. It should be noted that frozen section diagnosis of thyroid lesions can be extremely difficult, and most pathologists will see only a small number of thyroid cancers during their entire professional careers. As in few other situations, it is important that communication be clear between the pathologist and the surgeon as to how certain the histologic diagnosis is.[18] No doubt exists that the best way to insure this is for the pathologist to go to the operating room and obtain the specimen, do the frozen section, and return to the operating room to present his findings personally to the surgeon. If findings are doubtful, near total lobectomy should be carried out on the affected side and the isthmus resected. Further therapy, which may include subtotal lobectomy on the opposite side, may be instituted after permanent sections have clearly established a diagnosis of cancer. We have noted no increased morbidity or mortality from this practice in the past, and fortunately this situation has arisen much less frequently in recent years.

The third problem with the differentiated lesions, and especially the papillary cancers, is the increased malignancy in older men and women. It has been documented in several studies that the disease is much more lethal in women if it is first recognized when the patient is more than 40 years of age. In our unpublished series of over 270 cases of papillary cancer of the thyroid, the mortality from disease in patients followed for a minimum of 10 years was 8 percent in patients who were less than 40 when first treated and 30 percent in patients who were more than 40 when first treated. Over 80 percent of patients in our series who died from papillary carcinoma were over the age of 40 when first treated. This is puzzling to most workers in the field and makes us question both the reasons for this and our methods of treatment in the older age groups. We are interested in the role that the absence of female sex hormones might play in this trend toward greater malignancy in men and older women, but it will be many years before we can come to any conclusions. It is in this older age group that one finds a greater incidence of transformation of well differentiated thyroid cancers to the more malignant undifferentiated types, with both occurring in the same tumor. In these patients (about 6 to 8 percent in one study) the clinical course is usually typical of the more malignant variant. As a result of this, some surgeons (ourselves included) feel justified in pursuing a more aggressive approach to well differentiated thyroid cancers in the older age group even when the lesion is apparently small and intrathyroidal. In this situation we would be much more likely to consider a node dissection on the affected side in addition to our usual surgical treatment.

A fourth problem with this group of tumors is the presence of tumor dissemination within the gland and the prognostic significance of this finding. In the early 1950's the M. D. Anderson group[8, 22] discovered that serial section of the entire gland in patients with gross lesions in only one lobe revealed small tumor foci elsewhere in the gland in over 80 percent of cases. This finding resulted in the recommendation of total thyroidectomy in all cases of differentiated thyroid cancer, but when this was done, the incidence of complications was significantly increased, especially with respect to the development of permanent hypoparathyroidism. Surgical hypoparathyroidism is an extremely difficult condition to treat adequately and is a serious complication. As a result of this and because the long-term cure rate for the differentiated thyroid cancers was around 70 to 90 percent, even without the routine use of the more extensive resection, many surgeons questioned the need for total thyroidectomy. The practical solution to this problem has been to remove as much thyroid tissue as possible without causing hypoparathyroidism, which is accomplished by routine identification and preservation of as many parathyroid glands as possible, especially on the uninvolved or lesser involved side and by routinely employing subtotal lobectomy rather than total lobectomy on the uninvolved side. In the event that a parathyroid gland is identified at surgery after inadvertent removal, it can be sectioned thinly and implanted in the sternocleidomastoid muscle with some hope for continued function.

Recently some have advocated sparing most of the grossly uninvolved thyroid lobe (the involved side and the isthmus are excised), again because of the high cure rates with lesser procedures. We believe this is a mistake because we know that these lesions can be extremely slow growing and we know that microscopic foci are present in a high percentage of cases. We believe that to depend upon some hypothetical inhibition of further growth of these lesions by removal of the main tumor mass or on indefinite suppression by the use of thyroid hormone is unwarranted until we have a clearer understanding of the factors responsible for tumor inhibition.

A fifth problem arising with the differentiated thyroid cancers is that local invasion is a much more serious prognostic sign than is metastasis to neck nodes. Patients in whom the tumor invades the adjacent deep structures of the neck have a mortality risk four times as great as the patient in whom the primary tumor is not invasive. Of the 56 deaths from papillary cancer in our series, 20 occurred in patients with invasion of surrounding tissues. In the majority of these patients the tumor could not be excised completely. By contrast, patients who have lymph node metastases confined to the neck from well differentiated thyroid cancers have a prognosis only slightly less good than patients with intrathyroidal cancer, provided the nodal metastases can be removed by neck dissection. A classic example of the indolence of thyroid malignancy in neck nodes is seen in so-called lateral aberrant thyroid. The patient would present with a mass in the cervical lymphatic chain and a thyroid gland that was normal to palpation. The mass would be excised and found to be nearly normal-appearing thyroid tissue. After a period of several years many of the patients would present again with a clinically obvious thyroid malignancy. It took nearly two decades to clarify the malignant nature of lateral aberrant thyroid because some patients died of other causes before the primary became apparent and many others were lost to follow-up during the long disease-free interval.

In recent years the use of radical neck dissection has come under heavy criticism from the Cleveland Clinic group[9] on the basis that the jugular chain of nodes removed in the standard radical neck dissection is a secondary rather than a primary route of lymphatic drainage of the thyroid. They believe that in order to remove all the lateral cervical nodes en bloc, the carotid vessels would have to be sacrificed because some of the lateral cervical nodes lie deep to the carotids. They have repeatedly stressed the need for adequate central dissection because this is the region of primary lymphatic drainage. On the more conservative side of this question are those who have demonstrated unsuspected nodal metastases in up to 30 percent of patients who had prophylactic radical neck dissection during a period when that procedure was in vogue.[19] In our experience radical neck dissection has been very helpful, and we credit our high survival rates in patients with nodal metastases to its liberal use. At the present time we believe that the same beneficial effects can be obtained by using a modified radical neck dissection, sparing the sternocleidomastoid muscle when this can be accomplished without compromising the nodal dissection. There is continued debate on this issue within the surgical community, but we believe we should await longer follow-up studies from those centers where lesser procedures are advocated before adopting a less aggressive approach in the treatment of these tumors.

MEDULLARY CARCINOMA

Medullary carcinoma has been separated from the other thyroid carcinomas for several reasons.[2, 30] The pathologic criteria for this diagnosis are discussed in Chapter Four. Clinically it is the only thyroid tumor that is familial, although quite rare.[4] Also, it appears to be the only thyroid cancer that occurs with various other endocrinopathies, such as pheochromocytoma and hyperparathyroidism as well as carcinoid and neurofibromatosis. This has occurred in less than 15 percent of recorded cases. The survival rates (Table 10-6) are less than those for the differentiated carcinomas, with which medullary carcinoma was formerly grouped. It is important to realize that this tumor has metastasized to regional nodes at the time of original surgery in 50 to 67 percent of patients, and that node dissection, at least on the more involved side, is justified in nearly all cases if the primary tumor can be excised completely. It must be stressed that these lesions are hard to distinguish from the more undifferentiated thyroid cancers macroscopically, and frozen section diagnosis is mandatory in order that a more aggressive approach to the lesion can be taken at the initial operation. Medullary carcinomas and the metastatic lesions from them rarely take up radioactive iodine, so that when complete excision of tumor is doubtful, we would proceed with megavoltage external irradiation, which has given very good results in about 25 percent of treated cases, with most patients receiving at least some palliation.

The fact that many medullary carcinomas may secrete thyrocalci-

Table 10-6. Survival in Medullary Cancer of the Thyroid

Study	Stage	Survival Data	Number of Patients
Beahrs and Pasternak[2]	Confined to thyroid	85% 10-year survival	36
	with nodal metastases	42% 10-year survival	41
Hazard et al.[13]	All cases	30% mortality from diseases; all cases not followed for at least 10 years but some cases followed longer than 10 years; five patients (15%) died of other causes	21
Williams et al.[30]	All cases	33% mortality from diseases; all cases not followed for at least 10 years but some cases followed longer than 10 years; five patients (15%) died of other causes	

tonin in greatly increased amounts may prove to be of some diagnostic value as simpler means of determining serum thyrocalcitonin levels are developed.

UNDIFFERENTIATED TUMORS

The tumors in this group, the small cell and large cell undifferentiated carcinomas, are the most malignant of the thyroid cancers. They tend to occur in older age groups in sharp distinction to the differentiated thyroid cancers. Men and women are affected in equal proportion. The tumors are usually invasive at the time of operation and cannot be excised completely. They do not respond to suppressive therapy with thyroid extract. They will not concentrate radioactive iodine. As a rule, these lesions respond only transiently to megavoltage external radiation, if at all, but on occasion we have had an excellent response. Some of the recorded instances of cure of undifferentiated cancers by x-ray therapy have undoubtedly occurred in patients with medullary carcinomas which were formerly classified as small cell diffuse undifferentiated thyroid carcinomas with amyloid struma. Some of the five x-ray cures of small cell compact undifferentiated thyroid carcinomas reported by Smedal and Meissner[24] were said to have amyloid struma, the single most distinguishing feature of the medullary cancers, and these tumors are known to respond better to x-ray therapy than the true undifferentiated lesions. Also, there have been occasional instances of lymphoma presenting as primary thyroid tumor and initially misclassified as undifferentiated thyroid cancer in which dramatic x-ray response had led to review of the pathology with subsequent reclassification as lymphoma. If a lymphoma is misclassified it is usually called a small cell compact thyroid cancer, and the patient is usually younger than the typical elderly person who has undifferentiated thyroid cancer. As a general rule, surgical therapy of these lesions should be more radical when they are found incidentally than when the patient presents with symptoms referable to the tumor. Nearly all patients in this latter group are dead within a few months, so that biopsy and a short intensive course of external radiotherapy to check for tumor regression (in which case, a full course of radiotherapy is given) are all that is indicated. On the other hand, a small focus of tumor that is not invading the surrounding tissues is treated by near total thyroidectomy, and serious consideration is given to cervical node dissection on the side of the lesion or mediastinal node dissection if the lesion is low lying and central when there is the slightest suspicion of nodal metastases. In a good-risk patient with a small lesion in which the frozen section diagnosis is reasonably certain, we feel justified in proceeding with node dissection for prognostic purposes. After operation, these patients are given a 6,000 rads course of megavoltage external radiation to the neck. Most of the long-term survivors of this highly malignant disease are from this group.

REFERENCES

1. Attie, J. N.: The use of radioactive iodine in the evaluation of thyroid nodules. Surgery 47:611–622 (April) 1960.
2. Beahrs, O. H., and Pasternak, B. M.: Cancer of the thyroid gland. Curr. Probl. Surg. 3:1–38 (Dec.) 1969.
3. Black, B. M., YaDeau, R. E., and Wollner, L. B.: Surgical treatment of thyroidal carcinomas. Arch. Surg. 88:610–618 (April) 1964.
4. Block, M. A., Horn, R. C., Miller, J. M., et al.: Familial medullary cancer of the thyroid. Ann. Surg. 166:403–412 (Sept.) 1967.
5. Buckwalter, J. A.: Age and thyroid carcinoma. Arch. Surg. 82:916–924 (June) 1961.
6. Buckwalter, J. A., and Thomas, C. G., Jr.: Selection of surgical treatment for well-differentiated thyroid carcinomas. Ann. Surg. 176:565–578 (Oct.) 1972.
7. Cattell, R. B.: Indications for neck dissection in carcinoma of the thyroid. J. Clin. Endocr. 10:1099–1107 (Sept.) 1950.
8. Clark, R. L., Jr., White, E. C., and Russell, W. O.: Total thyroidectomy for cancer of thyroid: Significance of intraglandular dissemination. Ann. Surg. 149:858–866 (June) 1959.
9. Crile, G., Jr.: The fallacy of the conventional radical neck dissection for papillary carcinoma of the thyroid. Ann. Surg. 145:317–320 (March) 1957.
10. Crile, G., Jr.: Late results of treatment for papillary cancer of the thyroid. Ann. Surg. 160:178–182 (Aug.) 1964.
11. Frazell, E. F., and Foote, F. W., Jr.: Papillary cancer of the thyroid: A review of 25 years' experience. Cancer 11:895–922 (Sept.-Oct.) 1958.
12. Gottlieb, J. A., and Hill, C. S., Jr.: Chemotherapy of thyroid cancer with adriamycin: Experience with 30 patients. New Engl. J. Med. 290:193–197 (Jan. 24) 1974.
13. Hazard, J. B., Hawk, W. A., and Crile, G., Jr.: Medullary (solid) carcinoma; A clinicopathological entity. J. Clin. Endocr. 19:152–161 (Jan.) 1959.
14. Hedinger, E. (ed.): Thyroid Cancer. Conference on Thyroid Cancer, May, 1968. Victor Monograph Series No. 12. Berlin, Springer-Verlag, 1969.
15. Hirabayashi, R. N., and Lindsay, S.: Carcinoma of the thyroid gland: A statistical study of 390 patients. J. Clin. Endocr. 21:1596–1610 (Dec.) 1961.
16. Klopp, C. T., Rosvoll, R. V., and Winship, T.: Is destructive surgery ever necessary for treatment of thyroid cancer in children? Ann. Surg. 165:745–751 (May) 1967.
17. Lindsay, S., and Chaikoff, I. L.: The effects of irradiation on the thyroid gland with particular reference to the induction of thyroid neoplasms. Cancer Res. 24:1099–1107 (Aug.) 1964.
18. Meissner, W. A., and Adler, A.: Papillary carcinoma of the thyroid: A study of the pathology in 226 cases. A.M.A. Arch. Path. 66:518–525 (Oct.) 1958.
19. Meissner, W. A., Colcock, B. P., and Achenbach, H.: The pathologic evaluation of radical neck dissection for carcinoma of the thyroid. J. Clin. Endocr. 15:1432–1436 (Nov.) 1955.
20. Pochin, E. E.: Prospects from the treatment of thyroid carcinoma with radioiodine. Clin. Radiol. 18:113–125 (April) 1967.
21. Pochin, E. E.: Thyroid cancer: Treatment: Radioiodine therapy. In Werner, S. C., and Ingbar, S. H. (eds.): The Thyroid. 3rd ed. New York, Harper and Row, 1971, pp. 467–475.
22. Russell, W. O., Ibanez, M. L., Clark, R. L., et al.: Thyroid carcinoma. Classification, intraglandular dissemination, and clinicopathological study based upon whole organ sections of 80 glands. Cancer 16:1425–1460 (Nov.) 1963.
23. Silliphant, W. M., Klinck, G. H., and Leutin, M. S.: Thyroid carcinoma and death: A clinicopathological study of 193 autopsies. Cancer 17:513–525 (April) 1964.
24. Smedal, M. I., and Meissner, W. A.: The results of x-ray treatment in undifferentiated carcinoma of the thyroid. Radiology 76:927–935 (June) 1961.
25. Sutton, J. P., McSwain, B., and Diveley, W. L.: Carcinoma of the thyroid. Ann. Surg. 167:839–846 (June) 1968.

26. Thomas, C. G.: Dependency of thyroid cancer: A review. Ann. Surg. 146:879–891 (Dec.) 1957.
27. Tollefsen, H. R., and DeCosse, J. J.: Papillary carcinoma of the thyroid. The case for radical neck dissection. Am. J. Surg. 108:547–551 (Oct.) 1964.
28. Tollefsen, H. R., DeCosse, J. J., and Hutter, R. V. P.: Papillary carcinoma of the thyroid. A clinical and pathological study of 70 fatal cases. Cancer 17:1035–1044 (Aug.) 1964.
29. Veith, F. J., Brooks, J. R., Grigsby, W. P., et al.: The nodular goiter and cancer. A practical approach to the problem. New Engl. J. Med. 270:431–436 (Feb. 27) 1964.
30. Williams, E. D., Brown, C. L., and Doniach, I.: Pathological and clinical findings in a series of 67 cases of medullary carcinoma of the thyroid. J. Clin. Path. 19:103–113 (March) 1966.
31. Winship, T., and Rosvoll, R. V.: Childhood thyroid carcinoma. Cancer 14:734–743 (July-Aug.) 1961.
32. Winship, T., and Rosvoll, R. V.: Thyroid carcinoma in childhood: Final report on a 20 year study. Clin. Proc. Child. Hosp. 26:327–348 (Dec.) 1970.

Chapter Eleven

ANESTHESIA FOR THYROID SURGERY

Morris J. Nicholson, M.D.
and
Joseph P. Crehan, M.D.

HISTORY

The superficial location of the thyroid gland in the neck has for centuries made some of its pathologic states obvious to the lay public and a challenge to the medical profession. Patients with a swelling in the neck, commonly referred to as goiter, have sought relief because of suffocation, difficulty in swallowing, failure of the heart, or distressing disfigurement.

From the viewpoint of the medical historian, the role of anesthesia in the development of modern thyroid surgery is but one of the confusing aspects of the total picture which Halsted so aptly described in "The Operative Story of Goitre; The Author's Operation."[14]

Documented operations, admittedly few in number, were performed without anesthesia before the advent of ether, in 1846, and chloroform in 1847. Even the introduction of these two general anesthetic agents did not cause a great change in thyroid surgery, for as Halsted recounted:[14] "From 1880 to 1886, the period of my surgical activities in New York, I neither saw nor heard of an operation for goitre, except that in one instance I assisted Dr. Henry B. Sands to extirpate a small tumor from the right lobe of the thyroid gland. The patient, a male, was operated upon in the sitting posture, with a rubber bag to catch the blood tied about his neck. We had only two artery forceps, all, probably, that the hospital afforded, and these were of the mouse-tooth or bulldog variety (Liston's).'

Little mention is made of the anesthetic agents or methods used for the relatively small number of thyroid operations performed in the last half of the 19th century. We do know that in 1876 Clover of England introduced a method for the clinical administration of nitrous oxide with ether.[7] By 1892 Hewitt and White[16] had developed a gas machine for the controlled administration of nitrous oxide and oxygen. It can be assumed that the pioneer thyroid surgeons of Europe, England, and the United States employed some general anesthesia for pain relief during this time.

Following Koller's discovery[19] in 1884 of the ability of cocaine to produce topical anesthesia, Halsted,[13] in 1885, introduced the use of cocaine for regional nerve block anesthesia. Einhorn's[11] discovery of procaine in 1904, and its rapid acceptance for the production of local infiltration and regional block anesthesia, had a real impact on thyroid surgery. Soon thyroid operations were being performed under local infiltration and, in some instances, deep cervical plexus nerve block in all surgically advanced countries by a small number of pioneer surgeons.

In 1908 Crile[8,9] described his now historically important "anoci-association" technique of combining procaine infiltration with nitrous oxide inhalation anesthesia.

The 50-year period of 1920 to 1970 has been characterized by an explosion of newer knowledge regarding thyroid disease—its diagnosis, treatment (medical and surgical), and anesthetic care. It will suffice to list the pertinent developments in anesthesia during this period, the accumulative effects of which are now providing benefits for all patients undergoing thyroid surgery.

1920—Magill: Clinical development of endotracheal anesthesia.[28]

1922—Labat: Book on regional anesthesia.[20]

1923—Luckhardt and Carter: Discovery of ethylene.[25]

1923—Waters: Development of soda lime for carbon dioxide absorption.[40]

1926—Butzengeiger: Demonstration of the clinical use of avertin as a rectal anesthetic.[5]

1928—Sword: Introduction of the closed circle carbon dioxide absorption method of administering general anesthetic agents.[39]

1928—Henderson and Lucas: Demonstration of the anesthetic properties of cyclopropane.[15]

1930—Waters and Schmidt: Introduction of cyclopropane anesthesia to clinical practice.[41]

1931—Lundy: Nembutal (pentobarbital sodium) as an intravenous anesthetic agent.[26]

1934—Lundy: Introduction of sodium pentothal for the production of intravenous anesthesia.[27]

1942—Griffith and Johnson: Introduction of muscle relaxants into clinical anesthesia.[12]

1951-1956—Suckling,[38] Raventos,[34] and Johnstone[18]: Introduction of the fluorinated hydrocarbons into anesthesia practice.

1961-1963—Janssen: Introduction of drugs and the concept of neuroleptanalgesia into clinical anesthesia practice.[17]

Since 1920 the development of satisfactory anesthesia for thyroid surgery at the Lahey Clinic has evolved gradually.[37] The anesthetic agents have been changed repeatedly, and the methods of administration have been modified and improved.

General anesthesia is our choice for all thyroid operations because it fulfills the average patient's desire to be asleep and is relatively safe. In addition, it gives the surgeon the freedom he needs to accomplish the wide lateral exposure so essential for the radical removal of the thyroid gland without injury to the recurrent laryngeal nerves and the parathyroid glands. The carbon dioxide absorption method of administration is employed for these thyroid operations with endotracheal intubation as indicated.

A discussion of the role of the anesthesiologist in the management of the thyroid patient should include the preoperative preparation of the patient, premedication, selection of the anesthetic agent and method, and the management of operative and postoperative complications.

PREOPERATIVE PREPARATION OF THE PATIENT

The use of the potent and effective antithyroid agents (thiouracil, thiobarbital, propylthiouracil, methylthiouracil, and methimazole[1, 2, 24]) has revolutionized the anesthetic management of the patient with thyrotoxicosis. The indications for multiple-stage operations have shown a striking decline. The operative course is seldom fraught with danger, and postoperative reactions, when seen, are seldom severe.[1, 24]

Since one cannot assume that the proper responses will always follow the use of these agents, each patient should be evaluated carefully and treated until all signs of toxicity have been abolished. Since this degree of perfection in the preoperative management is at times difficult to obtain, the role of the anesthesiologist in the management of the thyroid patient must be stressed.

The preoperative preparation of the patient suffering from thyroid disease is the joint responsibility of the internist, the surgeon, and the anesthesiologist. From the medical standpoint, preparation should be directed toward the correction of the disturbed physiologic state caused by this systemic disease which affects practically every system of the body. The medical program must include rest, sedation, and a diet high in carbohydrates, protein, and vitamin content, plus the proper antithyroid medication. Hopefully these patients will be relieved of their presenting symptoms—nervousness, emotional instability, irritability, weight loss, weakness, increased appetite, intolerance to heat, dyspnea, palpitation, and, in the more severe cases, even vomiting and diarrhea.

Before the introduction of the antithyroid drugs it was thought necessary to prepare all patients with hyperthyroidism for surgery in the hospital (or at least at home) with bed rest. Since the introduction of

Table 11-1. Laboratory Values

Average serum thyroxine level in
    Hyperthyroid group — 22 mg. per 100 ml.
    Euthyroid group — 9 mg. per 100 ml.
    Hypothyroid group — 2 mg. per 100 ml.

Average ^{131}I uptake among
    Hyperthyroid group — 57 percent
    Euthyroid group — 9 percent
    Hypothyroid group — 6 percent
Serum thyroxine — 4.5 to 12.0 μg. per 100 ml.
Protein-bound iodine — 3.3 to 7.6 μg. per 100 ml.

these drugs, however, most patients can be prepared adequately and at the same time remain ambulatory. When thyrotoxic patients are prepared with antithyroid drugs, there is a progressive decrease of toxic signs and symptoms with an accompanying reduction in the basal metabolic rate and a fall in the serum protein-bound iodine and thyroxine levels (Table 11-1). It is not unusual for the patient with classic signs and symptoms of severe hyperthyroidism to come to operation after two months of preparation with a reduction of the basal metabolic rate from plus 65 to minus 10. Along with this amazing drop in the basal metabolic rate, the patient may present with signs of hypothyroidism. The clinical recognition of this state of hypometabolism is of real significance to the anesthesiologist. No longer do these patients require heavy preanesthetic medication, basal narcosis, and heavy postoperative sedation. After an intensive period of preparation with antithyroid drugs, they may be myxedematous and should have light premedication, no basal narcosis, light anesthesia for the operation, and light postoperative sedation. Failure to appreciate fully this great change in the metabolic activity associated with antithyroid agents may result in overmedication and undue depression if the anesthesiologist considers these patients in the light of their former toxic state rather than their actual state of hypometabolism.

Despite the highly desirable beneficial effects which usually follow the use of antithyroid drugs, it is important to note certain conditions which make for a guarded prognosis:

1. Age: 50 years or more.
2. Duration of the disease: more than one year.
3. Loss of one fifth or more of body weight.
4. Failure to gain weight during the preoperative period of rest and medication.
5. Failure of the pulse rate to drop to 100 or below during preparation.
6. Persistent auricular fibrillation or a history of previous cardiac failure.[22,23,36]

7. High initial basal metabolic rate and serum protein-bound iodine, and failure of these determinations to respond sufficiently under treatment.

8. Failure of preanesthetic medication to produce the expected sedation.

These danger signs may be found in any patient with severe primary hyperthyroidism and should always be appreciated.

The risk presented by patients suffering from the apathetic type of thyrotoxicosis is not so generally recognized because of failure to elicit these danger signs.[21] Most of these patients are elderly, have had the disease a long time, and have considerable weight loss. The signs of thyroid toxicity, restlessness, and agitation have long since become masked. The patient appears to be calm, the pulse rate may be slow, the basal metabolic rate only slightly elevated, and the serum protein-bound iodine almost normal. Unless this hidden toxicity is recognized and a careful regimen of bed rest, sedation, diet, and antithyroid medication is instituted, thyroidectomy may be hazardous and life threatening. Death may occur in these patients without any sign of a relighting of the thyroid activity such as that seen in patients with the activated type of hyperthyroidism.

All patients who are candidates for thyroidectomy should have a roentgenogram of the chest. If an intrathoracic extension or malignant condition is present or suspected, special x-ray films of the trachea should be obtained. Vocal cord function should be checked by indirect laryngoscopy in all patients who have formerly had thyroid operations, in those suspected of having malignant disease, and in those who demonstrate or complain of voice changes.

After the patient has been prepared adequately for operation by the internist and surgeon, he should be visited preoperatively by the anesthesiologist. This preanesthetic visit is quite important. Many times a patient will say he has no fear of the operation but is in truth afraid of the anesthetic. A preoperative visit can be valuable in allaying this fear and in gaining the patient's confidence. In addition, the anesthesiologist, by reviewing and evaluating the history, physical findings, laboratory data, and preoperative course, can better evaluate the physical state of the patient and anticipate problems that may arise during induction and maintenance of anesthesia, or in the postoperative period.

In our plan of preoperative preparation, we have never used the so-called sneak operation.

PREOPERATIVE MEDICATION

Preoperative medication should be given to relieve anxiety, to allay fear, and to make the patient less aware of his unaccustomed surroundings. The medication will do this to a limited degree, but equally important is the preanesthetic visit and reassurance by the anesthesiologist. A short discussion as to what will take place on arrival in the operating room and management during the patient's stay in the recovery room is extremely worthwhile. With the accomplishment of these objectives, the patient is usually calm, drowsy, and amnesic.[33]

Our routine medication consists of a combination of narcotics and a sedative, the doses of which are varied according to the age, vigor, and metabolic activity of the patient. Morphine sulfate, 8 to 10 mg., and scopolamine hydrobromide, 0.4 mg., are usually administered intramuscularly along with pentobarbital sodium, 100 mg. orally 1 1/2 hours before operation. The former is a metabolic depressant while the latter promotes amnesia, intensifies the narcosis of the morphine, depresses salivary secretion, and tends to offset somewhat the respiratory depression of morphine. Pentobarbital sodium (Nembutal), 100 mg., or in unusual cases, 200 mg., may be administered at bedtime the night before to provide a good night's sleep.

SELECTION OF THE ANESTHETIC AGENT AND METHOD

Two factors make anesthesia for thyroid operations different from most other types of anesthesia; they are the toxicity of the patient, and the possibility of respiratory obstruction occurring during the operation. Manipulation of the trachea during the operation may cause partial or complete respiratory obstruction. A single large adenoma may displace and compress the trachea. A large bilateral adenomatous goiter may narrow the trachea. Intrathoracic extensions of the thyroid gland are especially likely to cause obstruction during their extraction. A malignant tumor of the thyroid may cause obstruction because of its size, position, or even by direct invasion of the trachea. Acute laryngeal obstruction may occur during or after an operation when one or both recurrent laryngeal nerves have been injured.

Generally too much stress is placed upon the selection of the anesthetic agent and not enough on fundamental principles such as maintenance of an adequate airway and avoidance of anoxia. Our experience has shown the wisdom of electing the endotracheal method of anesthesia to ensure a free airway during most thyroid operations. However, it is essential that endotracheal intubation be employed for patients with (1) a deviated or compressed trachea, (2) recurrent hyperthyroidism, (3) cancer of the thyroid, (4) intrathoracic goiter, and (5) unilateral or bilateral paralysis of the vocal cords.[4, 30, 31]

Endotracheal intubation may become necessary during the course of the operation when the ordinary adjuvants, such as elevation of the chin, use of oral and nasal pharyngeal airways, light positive pressure on the breathing bag, and addition of helium to thin the mixture, fail to relieve satisfactorily the existing partial obstruction. A patient with a receding chin and a long epiglottis that falls back against the posterior pharyngeal wall to block the glottic opening on inspiration is likely to have breathing difficulty when the shoulders are elevated or when traction is made on the thyroid gland.

A small percentage of patients with cancer of the thyroid, adenomatous goiter with compression and deviation of the trachea, or large intrathoracic goiters will have persistent preoperative respiratory stridor. Such patients should be treated with great care, since muscular relaxation and even small amounts of premedication may lead to further respiratory embarrassment and the establishment of a vicious circle of hypoxia and narcosis. Light general anesthesia is even more dangerous, because it often causes sudden and more complete obstruction to take place. When such a pathologic condition is present, intubation under topical anesthesia is one of the most gratifying procedures in the practice of anesthesia. Once the endotracheal tube is in place and the stridor and the struggle to breathe have been relieved, these patients frequently fall asleep. After the intubation has been accomplished, general anesthesia may be instituted with impunity.

Most of our patients who are candidates for thyroid operations arrive in the operating suite in a calm and relaxed state of mind following the premedication, which has been administered 1 1/2 hours before the scheduled time of operation. While they are in the waiting room an intravenous infusion, usually consisting of 1,000 ml. of 5 percent dextrose and water or lactated Ringer's solution, is started, using an 18-gauge Teflon plastic needle that is inserted into one of the large veins in the left forearm. The legs are covered with elastic stockinette up to the knees and an appropriate headdress is applied to confine the hair. The patient is then taken to the operating room, placed on the operating table, and precordial leads are applied in order that cardiac monitoring may be carried out throughout the operation. A blood pressure cuff is applied and the preoperative blood pressure and pulse rate are obtained (Fig. 11–1).

Induction is generally accomplished by the injection of thiopental, 300 to 400 mg. of a 2 percent solution, into the intravenous tubing while the patient is being ventilated with 50 percent nitrous oxide and oxygen. Then succinylcholine, 40 to 50 mg., combined with decamethonium bromide, 3 to 4 mg., is injected and complete muscular relaxation is obtained. At this point an appropriate-sized endotracheal tube with inflatable cuff attached is introduced by direct laryngoscopy. The operating table is placed in a modified Fowler's position, and the appropriate-sized folded cloth support is placed under the shoulders to extend the neck. According to the anesthesiologist's preference, maintenance anesthesia may be provided by the addition of 1.0 to 1.5 percent halothane into a semiclosed system consisting of 1 liter of oxygen and 2 liters of nitrous oxide. Adequate ventilation is assured by assisting respiration. In our clinic, almost equally popular for maintenance anesthesia for these

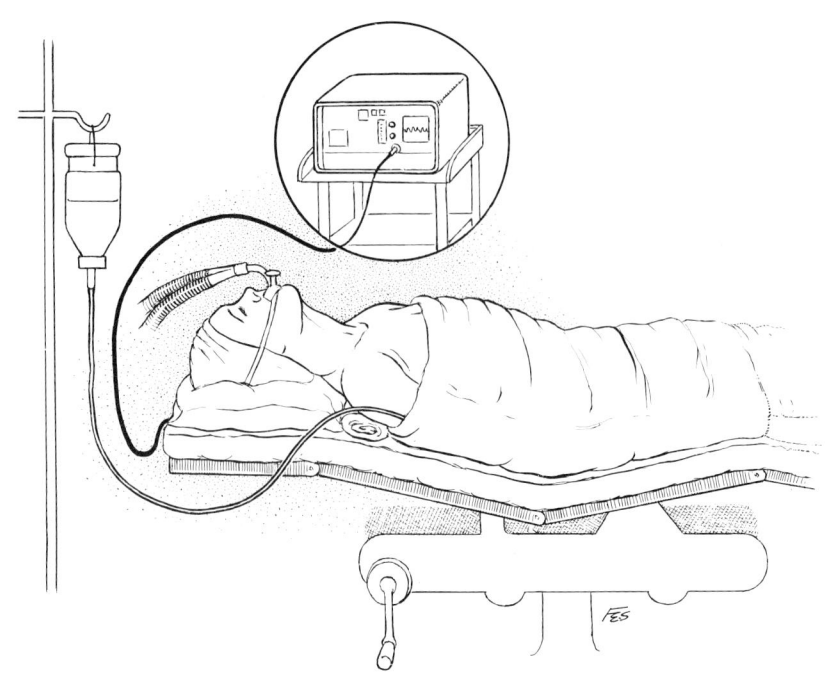

Figure 11-1. Position for thyroidectomy; modified Fowler's with shoulders elevated and head extended.

thyroid operations is the use of semiclosed nitrous oxide (oxygen) as described previously, with the judicious use of Innovar injected in 1 ml. increments up to a total of 5 ml. for the average operation. Should it seem necessary, small intermittent doses of thiopental may be added to this anesthetic regimen.

At the conclusion of the operation, the patient is extubated. When a satisfactory pattern of respiration has been established, he is moved to a bed which is placed in a modified Fowler's position. Postoperatively all thyroid patients remain in the recovery room until 8 a.m. the following day. During this time they are observed for possible respiratory difficulties and the wound is frequently inspected for swelling caused by hemorrhage. The intravenous fluids started in the operating room are continued and, if indicated, the cardiac monitoring may also be continued. Routinely, heated humidity (40 percent oxygen and 60 percent air) is used continuously by means of a Puritan face tent to provide additional inspired oxygen and to help to liquefy and mobilize retained secretions (Fig. 11-2).

Cyclopropane, which was used in many thousands of thyroid operations in the past, is seldom used now as we are somewhat concerned about the flammability of this explosive agent in the presence of the ever-increasing utilization of electrical apparatus. We are also more mindful of the inherent danger that lies in the apparent parasympathetic stimulating effects of cyclopropane which predispose to respiratory depression and cardiac arrhythmias.

Ether is seldom used, although it is an excellent agent, particularly well tolerated, and indicated in patients with asthma or any other type of bronchoconstrictive lung disease or heart trouble. But, like cyclopropane, ether and oxygen mixtures are flammable, and it is probably for this reason that this agent is not used more frequently.

MANAGEMENT OF OPERATIVE AND POSTOPERATIVE COMPLICATIONS

The ideal management of any complication is its anticipation and prevention. A member of the anesthesia department pays a preanesthetic visit to all patients the evening before the scheduled day of operation. Evaluation is made of the anesthetic risks that each patient presents and all positive information is recorded on his anesthesia sheet. Those patients presenting problems are discussed with members of the medical and surgical departments directly responsible for their preoperative preparation. When all this pertinent information is at hand, the preoperative medication is ordered, and the anesthetic agent and method are

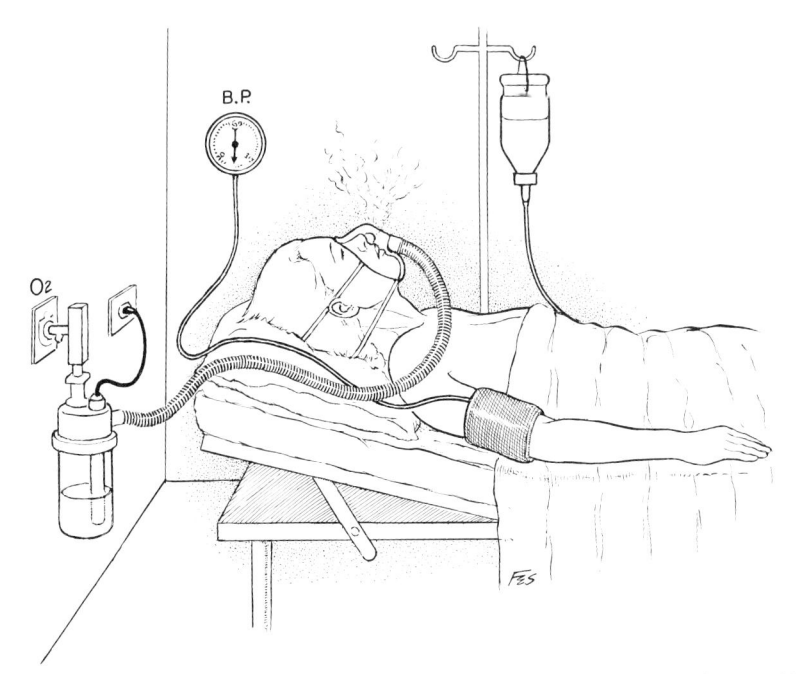

Figure 11-2. Postthyroidectomy position in recovery room. Semi-Fowler's position with heated nebulization via face mask.

chosen. Despite this careful evaluation, a certain unavoidable number of complications do occur. A discussion of their management by the anesthesiologist follows.

Hemorrhage

Hemorrhage is a serious potential hazard in all thyroid operations. Primarily a surgical complication, it is an important factor to be considered by the anesthesiologist. Patients with extremely large adenomatous goiters or cancer of the thyroid gland should be scheduled for a possible transfusion. If, during operation, bleeding seems to be excessive, steps should be taken to combat the inevitable blood pressure fall by the use of intravenous fluids or blood as indicated.

Hole in the Trachea

A hole in the trachea is a rare complication during thyroid surgery, but it is not uncommon during secondary thyroid operations. The anesthesiologist should recognize what has happened and increase the flow of gas so as to keep positive pressure in the trachea during all phases of respiration. The maintenance of positive pressure in the tracheobronchial tree throughout both inspiration and expiration prevents air or blood from being aspirated into the trachea while the surgeon closes the defect.

Carotid Sinus Syndrome

The carotid sinus syndrome is an infrequent but most alarming complication.[35] In our experience this syndrome has been seen most often in the elderly, arteriosclerotic, hypertensive patient. When pressure is applied at the bifurcation of the common carotid artery during the elevation of the skin flap or in an attempt to expose the superior thyroid arteries, one may see a sudden, severe, simultaneous drop in pulse rate, blood pressure, and respiration. Successful treatment depends on early recognition, interruption of the operation, and effective artificial respiration. When the precipitating influence has been removed, the patient's recovery is usually dramatic.

The injection of 5 to 10 ml. of 1 percent lidocaine solution around the bifurcation of the common carotid artery should be carried out immediately if the above-mentioned maneuvers have not already restored adequate circulation and respiration. In addition, the intravenous administration of a suitable vasopressor may be indicated. It is good practice to have the lidocaine solution on the table in a syringe whenever a radical neck dissection is contemplated or the removal of a carotid body tumor is anticipated. Under these conditions it is perhaps wise to infiltrate around the bifurcation of the common carotid artery, thus hopefully preventing this untoward reaction.

Postoperative Pulmonary Complications

Despite adequate preparation and careful surgical technique, postoperative complications do occur. Elevations of temperature, pulse, and respiration must be explained. Pain and discomfort may predispose to an ineffective cough, which could lead to atelectasis or pneumonia, or both.

Regurgitation and aspiration of stomach contents is another potential hazard, especially in the patient obtunded by narcotics, hypnotics, or tranquilizers. Pain should be relieved by appropriate dosage of narcotics or tranquilizers since a patient restless or struggling because of pain is potentially as hazardous as the one who is obtunded. The restless patient may dislodge vascular ties with resultant hemorrhage, while respiratory depression, inadequate ventilation, and associated problems may develop in the obtunded patient.

In an attempt to circumvent the problems associated with an absent or ineffective cough, warm oxygen-enriched mist is administered continuously for 48 hours to all patients. This will, hopefully, ease the discomfort and liquefy secretions so that they are more easily mobilized. If the patient cannot or will not cough effectively, the inhalation of ultrasonically nebulized sterile water is used to produce coughing.

Postoperative Respiratory Obstruction

Postoperative obstruction of the airway, partial or complete, is a serious, potentially lethal event that demands prompt attention. Most commonly precipitated by hemorrhage, the signs and symptoms of airway obstruction—swelling of the neck, inspiratory stridor, agitation or restlessness, as well as cyanosis, tachycardia, and cardiac arrhythmias—may develop slowly or rapidly. When due to arterial bleeding, the signs and symptoms develop rapidly. The increased pressure, being confined to a relatively small area, causes blood to penetrate and dissect tissue planes and produces venous obstruction and, ultimately, edema, particularly of the laryngopharynx and glottic opening. Since swelling may be massive and associated changes such as stridor and obstruction sudden, the diagnosis is usually evident. Venous bleeding, on the other hand, may be insidious, progressing over a period of hours with slowly developing signs and symptoms.

Whether the bleeding is arterial or venous, clinical judgment and experience alone will not guarantee an accurate appraisal of the degree of respiratory obstruction. This is properly evaluated only by indirect or direct laryngoscopy.

A useful clinical guideline to the patency of the laryngeal opening and proper functioning of the vocal cords is said to be the presence or absence of inspiratory stridor. When stridor is present, some degree of obstruction is evident. If absent, deductions or evaluations may be erroneous or misleading. Stridor results when a large volume of air at increased velocity impinges on a restricted orifice. On the other hand, quiet breathing of a low tidal volume at a reduced flow rate in the sedated patient does not always produce stridor. To properly evaluate such a patient, he should be stimulated to take a deep breath and, hopefully, phonate. If obstruction is present, stridor will be evident.

Inspiratory stridor means airway obstruction, either minimal or severe. The degree of obstruction can be evaluated properly only by laryngoscopy. Since the insertion of a laryngoscope or the application of a topical anesthetic may produce laryngeal spasm in this already compromised airway, with resulting complete obstruction, administration of a short-acting muscle relaxant before instrumentation is attempted should be considered. When inspection of the glottic area is undertaken, one must be prepared to insert an endotracheal tube. Thus, all necessary agents and equipment for artificial ventilation must be at hand.

Emergency opening of the wound will relieve pressure and can be a worthwhile maneuver, but this will not relieve the laryngeal obstruction resulting from edema.

Since the precipitating factor, hemorrhage, is properly controlled only by surgical intervention, it is logical to return the patient to the operating room. If time permits, no intervention is undertaken until the patient is prepared and draped and the surgical team is ready for any necessary procedure or assistance. The patient is then reanesthetized and the wound is reopened. Glottic edema may be of such magnitude that landmarks are obliterated and attempts at intubation are unsuccessful. Obviously, in such a situation, the alternative is rapid tracheotomy. If intubation is successful, the crisis is resolved, and the surgical procedure can be carried out in the customary elective manner.

In the hope of avoiding tracheotomy, the endotracheal tube may be left in place for a period of hours. Although edema may have a rapid onset, it subsides slowly. Although the cause, hemorrhage, is corrected, the insult, edema, remains. Leaving an endotracheal tube in place rather than performing a tracheotomy may be deceptive; a snug-fitting endotracheal tube may promote edema. If the patient is restless and objects to the tube, the possibility of the production of further edema is likely. Although occasional patients may be spared a tracheotomy by this conservative approach, we generally prefer to perform a tracheotomy.

TRACHEOTOMY

As mentioned, hemorrhage into the thyroid wound, marked edema of the false cords, or unilateral or bilateral cord paralysis may occur as postoperative complications following thyroid surgery, making tracheotomy necessary. The ideal place to perform a tracheotomy is in the operating room with the operative field and the surgical team ready before administration of the anesthetic is started. These patients are

ANESTHESIA FOR THYROID SURGERY

often dangerously near complete respiratory obstruction, and even the spraying of a topical anesthetic agent into the throat may produce laryngeal spasm. For this reason, no attempt to anesthetize the throat or to introduce an endotracheal tube under topical anesthesia should be made until the operating team is ready to proceed. This precaution is observed to allow for an immediate emergency tracheotomy should complete respiratory obstruction ensue during the establishment of anesthesia and before endotracheal intubation can be accomplished.

Once the endotracheal tube has been placed, the operation can be accomplished in a routine fashion. As shown in Figure 11-3, just before

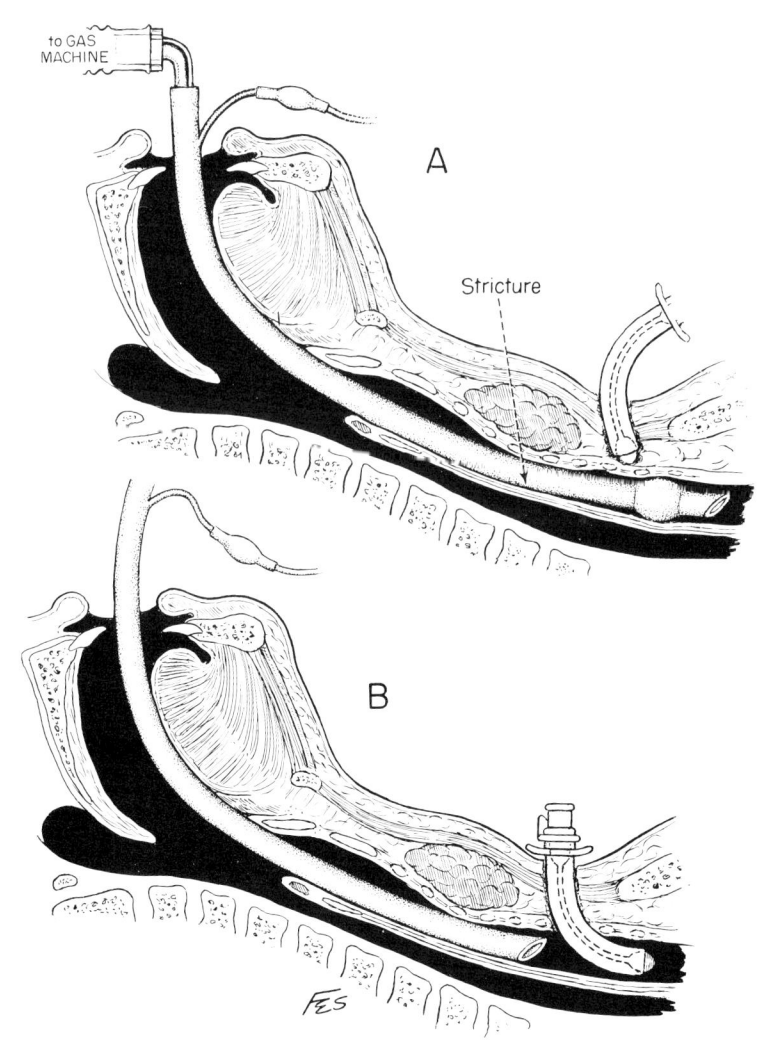

Figure 11-3. *A,* Endotracheal tube in place immediately before insertion of tracheotomy tube. *B,* Endotracheal tube withdrawn, allowing introduction of tracheotomy tube with occluding obturator permitting endotracheal anesthesia to be maintained.

the tracheotomy tube is inserted, the endotracheal tube is withdrawn to a point just proximal to the opening. If the obturator is left in the tracheotomy tube after its introduction, administration of the anesthetic agent can be continued until the operation has been completed.

Against the possibility that the patient may require postoperative mechanical ventilatory assistance, we prefer the use of a cuffed rubber tube readily adapted to a ventilating device by a standard connector. A constantly heated aerosol of sterile water is administered to all tracheotomized patients by means of a tracheotomy mask or a T-tube adapter. We believe this helps to maintain the proper ciliary action, prevents drying and encrustation, and aids in the liquefaction and, thus, the mobilization of retained secretions. With proper humidification of the inspired air, *suctioning of the trachea, with its inherent drawbacks and hazards, is seldom necessary.* Although the ability to generate rapid air flow may be reduced by tracheotomy, seldom will this interfere with mobilization and expulsion of liquefied secretions by coughing. There is no justification for the routine p.r.n. order for suctioning the trachea.

In the past, tracheotomy has been looked upon as a very formidable procedure and one that should be undertaken only in desperation. This attitude has caused this lifesaving procedure in some instances to be delayed unduly until irreparable damage has been done or a fatality has occurred. Dr. Lahey aptly summarized the situation concerning tracheotomy in the following statement, "If you are at a loss to know whether or not tracheotomy should be done, that is the time to do it, for further delay and procrastination may cost the patient his life." Tracheotomy may be done with facility and with very little discomfort to the patient and should not prolong his convalescence unduly. There should be no hesitancy in performing a tracheotomy on any patient who shows evidence of increasing postoperative respiratory obstruction.

ANESTHESIA FOR EMERGENCY SURGERY IN THE PRESENCE OF HYPERTHYROIDISM

When a patient with untreated or inadequately treated hyperthyroidism requires an emergency operation, a variety of questions must quickly be answered on clinical grounds.

1. What are the duration and severity of the hyperthyroidism? Are signs of impending thyrotoxic crisis present, such as great weight loss, significant fever, tachycardia of 120 beats per minute, loss of emotional control, overactivation, congestive heart failure, dyspnea, marked sweating, diarrhea, and jaundice?

2. Is the patient suffering from any of the conditions that have been known to precipitate thyrotoxic crisis, such as fever, pelvic inflammatory disease, appendicitis, acute cholecystitis, subacute bacterial endocarditis, diabetic acidosis, insulin reaction, digitalis withdrawal or intoxication, withdrawal of propylthiouracil or iodine, eclampsia, or pulmonary embolism?[29]

3. How much time can be spent treating the hyperthyroidism before the proposed operation is performed?

When the emergency treatment of hyperthyroidism is undertaken, emphasis must be placed on drugs—*reserpine, hydrocortisone, iodine,* and *propylthiouracil*.[6, 10] Therapy must proceed in three directions:

1. General measures to support nutrition by hydration with 2 to 3 liters of glucose in water or saline, oxygen to treat or forestall hypoxia; icepacks, alcohol sponges, or a refrigerated cooling blanket to combat hyperpyrexia.

2. Reserpine, 2.5 to 5 mg. intramuscularly and 2.5 mg. every 6 hours, to lessen the hyperactivity of the cardiovascular and central nervous system.

3. Corticosteroids to replace or reinforce adrenocortical function—hydrocortisone, 100 mg. intravenously, and cortisone acetate, 100 mg. intramuscularly every 3 hours.

4. To suppress the release of thyroxine from the thyroid gland, 1 to 3 gm. of sodium iodide should be added to the intravenous solution per day. In addition, propylthiouracil, 1 to 3 gm., should be administered orally each 24 hours to inhibit the production of thyroid hormones.

When as much preparation as the situation will permit has been accomplished, it is important that adequate preoperative sedation be provided. In addition to the customary morphine, atropine, and Nembutal, supplementary intravenous administration of Nembutal or Innovar should be considered.

When the contemplated operation lends itself to spinal anesthesia, this is our choice. Nevertheless, we also induce sleep with thiopental given intravenously and administer large flows of an equal mixture of nitrous oxide and oxygen.

Should the contemplated procedure require general anesthesia, we prefer heavy premedication and induction with thiopental. While maintaining ventilation with 50 percent nitrous oxide and 50 percent oxygen, a relaxing dose of succinylcholine chloride is administered, and intubation with a cuffed endotracheal tube is performed. Anesthesia is maintained with high flows of halothane, nitrous oxide, and oxygen. This technique helps to dissipate body heat and provides the high oxygen content so necessary for these patients.

No matter what type of anesthesia is administered, continuous cardiac and body temperature monitoring are essential in the operating and recovery rooms. In anticipation of the very real possibility of the development of fulminant hyperpyrexia, the patient should be on a cooling blanket, and procaine or procainamide should be available to treat the hyperpyrexia should it occur.[3, 32] During the postoperative period an intensive treatment regimen for hyperthyroidism must be continued.

REFERENCES

1. Astwood, E. B.: Treatment of hyperthyroidism with thiourea and thiouracil. J.A.M.A. 122:78–81 (May 8) 1943.
2. Bartels, E. C.: Propylthiouracil; its use in preoperative treatment of severe and complicated hyperthyroidism. West. J. Surg. 56:226–235 (April) 1948.
3. Beldavs, J., Small, V., Cooper, D. A., et al.: Postoperative malignant hyperthermia: A case report. Canad. Anaesth. Soc. J. 18:202–212 (March) 1971.
4. Boutros, A. R.: Anaesthesia and the thyroid gland: A review. Canad. Anaesth. Soc. J. 8:586–615 (Nov.) 1961.
5. Butzengeiger, O.: Klinische Erfahrungen mit Avertin (E 107). Deutsch. Med. Wschr. 53:712–713 (April 22) 1927.
6. Canary, J. J., Schaaf, M., Duffy, B. J., Jr., and Kyle, L. H.: Effects of oral and intramuscular administration of reserpine in thyrotoxicosis. New Eng. J. Med. 257:435–442 (Sept. 5) 1957.
7. Clover, J. T.: On an apparatus for administering nitrous oxide gas and ether, singly or combined. Brit. Med. J. 2:74–75 (July 15) 1876.
8. Crile, G. W.: Surgical aspects of Graves' disease with reference to the psychic factor. Ann. Surg. 47:864–869 (June) 1908.
9. Crile, G. W.: Nitrous oxide anaesthesia and a note on anoci-association, a new principle in operative surgery. Surg. Gynec. Obstet. 13:170–173 (Aug.) 1911.
10. Dillon, P. T., Babe, J., Meloni, C. R., et al.: Reserpine in thyrotoxic crisis. New Eng. J. Med. 283:1020–1023 (Nov. 5) 1970.
11. Einhorn, A., quoted by Braun, H.: Ueber einige neue örtliche anaesthetica (Stovain, Alypin, Novocain). Deutsch. Med. Wschr. 31:1667–1671 (Oct.) 1905.
12. Griffith, H. E., and Johnson, G. E.: The use of curare in general anesthesia. Anesthesiology 3:418–420 (July) 1942.
13. Halsted, W. S.: Practical comments on the use and abuse of cocaine. New York Med. J. 42:294–295 (Sept. 12) 1885.
14. Halsted, W. S.: The operative story of goitre; the author's operation. In Surgical Papers by William Stewart Halsted. Vol. 2. Baltimore, Johns Hopkins Press, 1924, pp. 257–423.
15. Henderson, V. E., and Lucas, G. H. W.: Cyclopropane; a new anesthetic. Anesth. Analg. 9:1–6 (Jan.–Feb.) 1930.
16. Hewitt and White, quoted by Keys, T. E.: The History of Surgical Anesthesia. With an Introductory Essay by Chauncey D. Leake, and a Concluding Chapter The Future of Anaesthesia by Noel A. Gillespie. New York, Henry Schuman, Inc., 1945.
17. Janssen, P. A.: [Comparative pharmacological data on 6 new basic 4'-fluorobutyrophenone derivatives: haloperidol, haloanisone, triperidol, methylperidine, haloperidide, and dipiperone. l.] Arzneimittelforsch 11:819–824 (Sept.) 1961.
18. Johnstone, M.: Human cardiovascular response to fluothane anaesthesia. Brit. J. Anaesth. 28:392–410 (Sept.) 1956.
19. Koller, C.: Vorläufige Mitthelung über Locale Anästhesing. Am Auge Klin. Monatsb. Augenh. Beilageheft 22:60–63, 1884.
20. Labat, G.: Regional Anesthesia: Its Technic and Clinical Application. Philadelphia, W. B. Saunders Company, 1922.
21. Lahey, F. H.: Non-activated (apathetic) type of hyperthyroidism. New Eng. J. Med. 204:747–748 (April 9) 1931.
22. Lahey, F. H., Bartels, E. C., Warren, S., and Meissner, W. A.: Thiouracil—its use in the preoperative treatment of severe hyperthyroidism. Surg. Gynec. Obstet. 81:425–439 (Oct.) 1945.
23. Lahey, F. H., and Hamilton, B. E.: Thyrocardiacs; their diagnostic difficulties; their surgical treatment. Surg. Gynec. Obstet. 39:10–14 (July) 1924.

24. Lahey, F. H., Hurxthal, L. M., and Driscoll, R. E.: Thyrocardiac disease: A review of 614 cases. Ann. Surg. 118:681–691 (Oct.) 1943.
25. Luckhardt, A. B., and Carter, J. B.: Ethylene as gas anesthetic. J.A.M.A. 80:1440–1442 (May 19) 1923.
26. Lundy, J. S.: Experience with sodium ethyl (1-methylbutyl) barbiturate (Nembutal) in more than 2,300 cases. Surg. Clin. N. Amer. 11:909–915 (Aug.) 1931.
27. Lundy, J. S.: Intravenous anesthesia: Preliminary report of the use of two new thiobarbiturates. Proc. Staff Meet. Mayo Clin. 10:536–543 (Aug. 21) 1935.
28. Magill, I. W.: Endotracheal anaesthesia. Proc. Roy. Soc. Med. 22:83–88 (Dec.) 1928.
29. McArthur, J. W., Rawson, R. W., Means, J. H., and Cope, O.: Thyrotoxic crisis: An analysis of 36 cases seen at Massachusetts General Hospital during the past 25 years. J.A.M.A. 134:868–874 (July 5) 1947.
30. Nicholson, M. J.: Anesthesia for thyroid surgery. Surg. Clin. N. Amer. 25:627–644 (June) 1945.
31. Nicholson, M. J.: Role of the anesthesiologist in the management of thyroid patients. Med. Rec. Ann. 47:385–394 (Jan.) 1953.
32. Nicholson, M. J.: Malignant hyperthermia with subsequent uneventful general anesthesia. Case History No. 65, with discussions by Mills, D. E., Marcy, J. H., Britt, B. A., and Zsigmond, E. K. Anesth. Analg. 50:1104–1112 (Nov.–Dec.) 1971.
33. Nicholson, M. J., and Crehan, J. P.: Preoperative preparation. In Hale, D. E. (ed.): Anesthesiology. 2nd ed. Philadelphia, F. A. Davis Co., 1963, pp. 179–208.
34. Raventos, J.: The action of fluothane; a new volatile anaesthetic. Brit. J. Pharm. 11:394–410 (Dec.) 1956.
35. Ruzicka, E. R., and Eversole, U. H.: The carotid sinus in anesthesiology: Report of two cases. Lahey Clin. Found. Bull. 3:47–54 (Oct.–Dec.) 1942.
36. Sise, L. F.: Anesthesia for thyrocardiac patients. J.A.M.A. 105:1662–1665 (Nov. 23) 1935.
37. Sise, L. F.: Development of anesthesia for thyroid surgery. In Frank Howard Lahey Birthday Volume. Springfield, Illinois, Charles C Thomas, 1940, pp. 419–424.
38. Suckling, C. W.: Some chemical and physical factors in the development of fluothane. Brit. J. Anaesth. 29:466–472 (Oct.) 1957.
39. Sword, B. C.: Closed circle method of administration of gas anesthesia. Anesth. Analg. 9:198–202 (Sept.–Oct.) 1930.
40. Waters, R. M.: Clinical scope and utility of carbon dioxide filtration in inhalation anesthesia. Anesth. Analg. 3:20–22 (Feb.) 1924.
41. Waters, R. M., and Schmidt, E. R.: Cyclopropane anesthesia. J.A.M.A. 103:975–983 (Sept. 29) 1934.

Chapter Twelve

SURGICAL TECHNIQUE

Cornelius E. Sedgwick, M.D.

The mortality rate of thyroidectomy as reported in several large series approaches zero. This can be accomplished only by a well performed standardized technique. The morbidity rate should be less than 5 percent. Morbidity consists of postoperative hemorrhage, wound infection, recurrent laryngeal nerve palsy, and postoperative hypoparathyroidism. A well executed thyroidectomy will keep this morbidity to a minimum. The step-by-step technique of thyroidectomy as described in this chapter was originally designed and advocated by Dr. Lahey. Over the years this technique has been only slightly modified by other surgeons of the Lahey Clinic. Although other methods have been mastered by thyroid surgeons with equally good results, our experience has been limited to this procedure. This method has stood the test of time (50 years) and numbers (over 40,000 patients). It is particularly recommended for the surgeon who has not yet standardized a satisfactory procedure. For the thyroid surgeon who has mastered other techniques it may be superfluous. The technique is easy to learn if special attention is paid to the details as outlined. It is the many details put together that make for a perfect result. At the Lahey Clinic literally hundreds of surgical fellows and residents have learned this technique and may attest to its excellence.

Surgery plays only one part in the successful treatment of thyroid disease. No matter how technically perfectly thyroidectomy is performed, if the patient is brought into the operation theater in either a hypothyroid or hyperthyroid state, disaster may follow. If the patient is a thyrocardiac the services of the cardiologist are mandatory. If the patient is euthyroid, but proper anesthesia is not available, complications may occur. If an expert in diagnosing thyroid pathology from a frozen section is lacking, the wrong procedure may be elected. For the best results, treatment of the thyroid patient demands the services not only of the surgeon but also of the internist, the cardiologist, the anesthesiologist, and the pathologist—all experienced with thyroid disease.

Anesthesia is discussed in Chapter Eleven.

SURGICAL TECHNIQUE 171

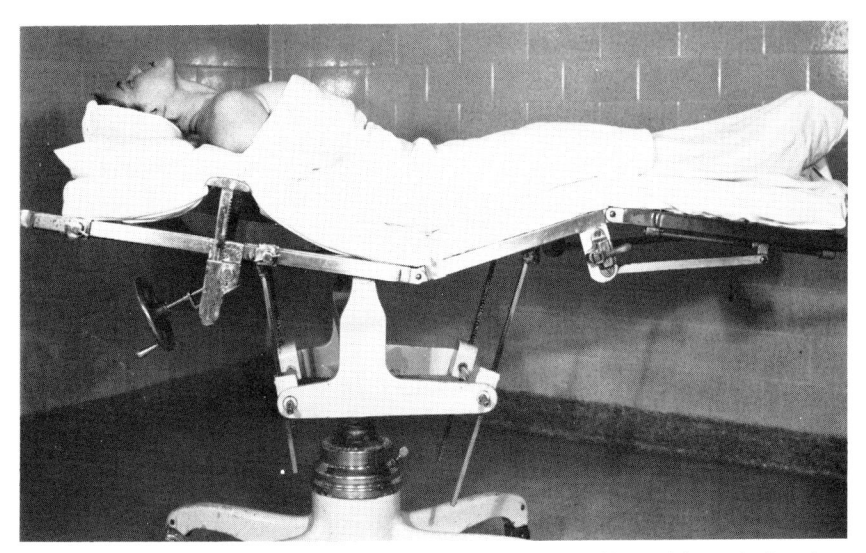

Figure 12-1. Position for patient. Note semisitting position with neck flexed to bring the thyroid forward.

POSITION ON THE OPERATING TABLE

The proper position and draping of the patient on the operating room table are important for maximum exposure (Fig. 12-1). The patient should be in a semisitting position. A bar or firm pillow is placed beneath the shoulders to allow maximum hyperflexion of the neck. Surgical drapes should be applied so that the entire anterior aspect of the neck from the chin to the suprasternal notch is exposed.

TECHNIQUE OF THYROIDECTOMY

Anterior Exposure of the Thyroid Gland

The Incision

The thyroid scar may be the only lasting objective evidence to the patient who has recovered from thyroidectomy. A conspicuous scar as the result of a poorly planned and designed incision, particularly in women, may be distressing. Long after recovery from the operation and the symptoms of thyroid disease, an ugly scar, because of its prominent location constantly exposed in the neck, may be a serious source of embarrassment to both patient and surgeon. Indeed, many women are more concerned preoperatively about the resultant scar than the actual surgery.

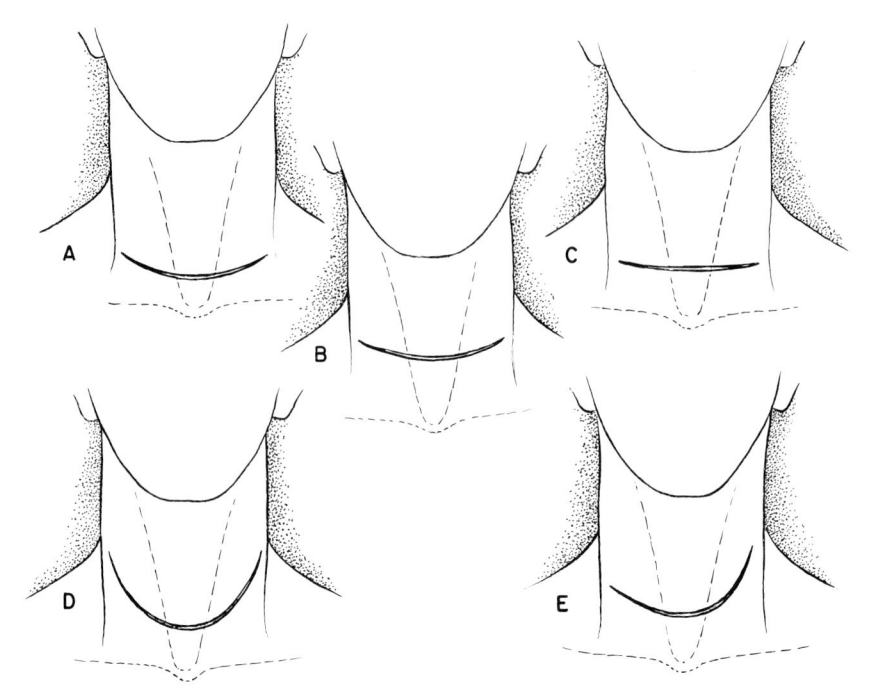

Figure 12-2. Skin incision for thyroidectomy. *A,* Proper—symmetrical curve at proper level. *B,* Too high—cannot be concealed. *C,* Too straight with inadequate curve—does not fall into folds between neck and chest. *D,* Too much of horseshoe type—does not permit concealment. *E,* Asymmetrical skin of right side has slipped down over front of chest. Had compensatory elevation of the incision been made (right side), it would have descended to the proper level.

A proper incision should have two features: (1) a well planned and designed incision to provide as much concealment as possible, and (2) an incision long enough so that the skin flap can be elevated for adequate exposure of the thyroid gland.

We prefer a low collar incision with a gentle curve upward (Fig. 12-2). It should be placed at a level at which a necklace will naturally rest to conceal the incision. If placed too high it is constantly visible. It must not be straight but rather curved upward to disappear between the folds of the neck and the chest. A common mistake that produces a more conspicuous scar is the horseshoe-type of incision in which the lateral limbs run too high and can never be concealed. The incision must be symmetrical, extending the same distance on each side from the midline; it must not be unbalanced, that is, one side higher than the other, because this will make it more noticeable. Many times the incision must be planned according to the size and shape of the goiter. A unilateral enlargement of the thyroid requires that the limb of the incision over the enlarged lobe be at a higher level. Once the enlarged lobe is removed, the skin will slip downward to produce a balanced, symmetrical scar. Over a large and prominent goiter the skin incision must be placed higher than normal. Once the stretched skin is relieved by removal of the goiter it will then descend to the proper level. The surgeon who gives attention to these few simple details regarding the thyroid incision will be well rewarded many times over by the satisfaction of his patients.

Elevation of the Flap

The skin, subcutaneous fat, and platysma are elevated as one layer. The fascial plane between the posterior sheath of the platysma and the sheath of the sternohyoid muscle is relatively avascular and permits the flap to be raised with little, if any, bleeding. To find this plane for dissection requires attention to almost subtle details and is well worth the effort. In well developed men the platysma is prominent; in obese women its fibers are not easily recognized in the subcutaneous fat. The platysmal fibers are most easily identified at the lateral margin of the incision. After the skin incision has been completed, the platysma muscle is identified laterally and its fibers divided, exposing the fascia of the prethyroid muscles (the sternohyoid and the sternothyroid; Fig. 12–3). If the bared muscle fibers of the prethyroid muscle are exposed, the dissection has passed through the desired fascial plane. As the surgeon approaches the midline, dividing the platysma, it will disappear. At this site the subcutaneous fat is divided, exposing the fascia of the prethyroid muscles over which lie the superficial veins. The superficial veins are not elevated with the flap and thus they act as a deep landmark to keep the proper fascial plane. Avoiding injury to the superficial veins prevents unnecessary bleeding. Leaving the midline, the surgeon continues the dissection toward the opposite side, exposing and dividing the platysma. The flap with skin, platysma, and subcutaneous tissue is now ready for elevation.

By applying upward traction, the flap is raised well above the thyroid notch by a combination of sharp and blunt dissection in a rela-

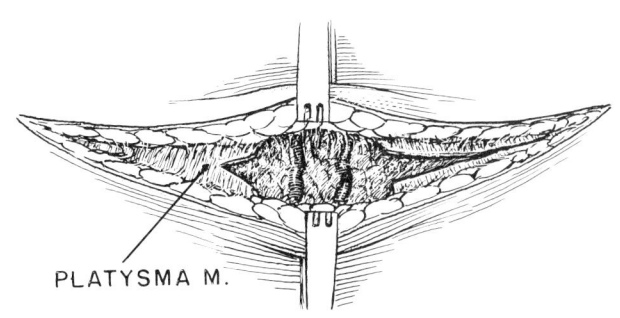

Figure 12–3. Division of platysma. Platysma fibers well visualized laterally. Medial—fat has been excised with flap. Superficial veins and fascia are seen over prethyroid muscles.

tively avascular plane. At the upper aspect of this dissection the flap appears to adhere more securely to the underlying fascia. If the flap is first raised in the midline, then laterally, the area between presents as a fibrous band interwoven with vessels running between the subcutaneous fat and the deeper structures. This fibrous tissue together with the vessels may be ligated and divided, allowing the flap to be sufficiently pushed upward (Fig. 12-4). One of the most important technical steps in thyroidectomy is high elevation of the flap. The flap can be elevated satisfactorily only before the prethyroid muscles are divided. Failure to do so at this time will compromise the all-important feature of anatomical exposure. Occasionally, if the goiter is low-lying or to allow better skin closure, the lower flap may be freed from the underlying fascia down to the level of the suprasternal notch.

Division of the Prethyroid Muscles (The Sternohyoid and the Sternothyroid)

Although this maneuver is not universally accepted, the prethyroid muscles should be divided in all cases to obtain adequate exposure and to perform a thyroidectomy safely. If the muscles are severed high, preserving their innervation from the descending branch of the ansa hypoglossal nerve which enters the muscle low, and are later carefully

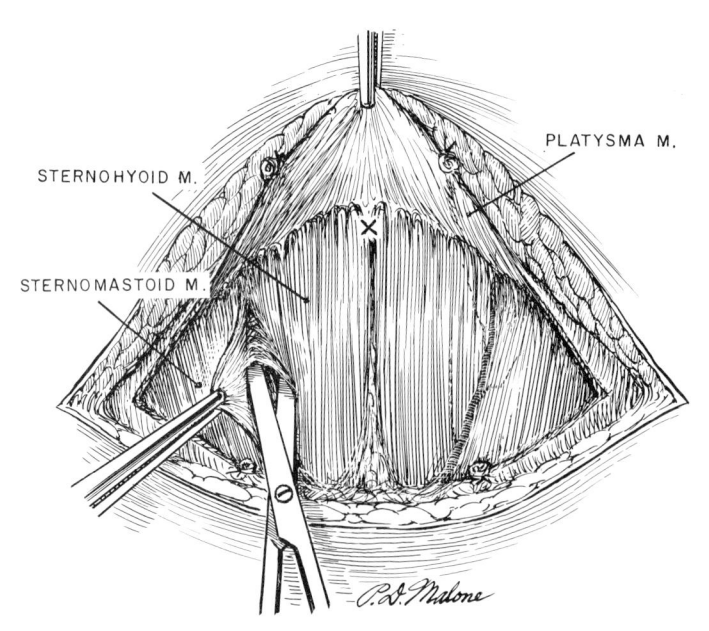

Figure 12-4. Elevation of flap, X, high to above thyroid notch. Fascia being divided between medial border of sternocleidomastoid muscle and lateral border of strap muscles (right side).

sutured, no disability or disfigurement results. Disfiguring atrophy of the prethyroid muscles, with the sunken neck and prominent trachea, is the result of dividing the prethyroid muscles and their innervation too low in the neck.

The prethyroid muscles are mobilized for transection by freeing their lateral and medial fascial attachments (Fig. 12–4). The fascia of the lateral border of the sternohyoid is attached to the fascia of the medial anterior border of the sternocleidomastoid muscle. If this fascia between the two muscles is divided along the medial edge of the sternocleidomastoid muscle, the anterior jugular vein will be spared, and the communicating veins between the anterior jugular and external jugular veins can easily be visualized, ligated, and divided. The medial borders of the sternohyoid and sternothyroid muscles are best identified in the midline low in the neck. The midline of the trachea above the suprasternal notch should be determined by palpation and this area explored. Often a small amount of free fatty tissue is a clue to the midline (Fig. 12–5 A). The finding of the midline before the midline fascia is divided is important in order to visualize, ligate, and divide the communicating veins crossing the midline from the anterior jugular of one side to the anterior jugular of the other.

With the borders of the prethyroid muscle mobilized by blunt dissection, their posterior sheaths are separated from the underlying thyroid capsule. This procedure is accomplished better and bleeding is avoided if it is started over the lower section of the thyroid rather than in the region of the upper poles. A common error is to separate only the sternohyoid and leave the sternothyroid attached to the thyroid capsule. This is particularly true in hyperplastic glands, as found in Graves' disease. A pericapsular reaction seems to occur so that the sternothyroid adheres to the capsule of the thyroid gland. This may be avoided by first elevating the sternohyoid and then carefully looking for the medial border of the sternothyroid, which is more lateral and in an enlarged gland may appear as the capsule of the thyroid itself (Fig. 12–5 B). If the operator is aware of this situation, he identifies the sternothyroid and elevates it from the capsule. Both prethyroid muscles are then separated from the gland by blunt dissection. While the medial border of the sternocleidomastoid is retracted downward and outward by the assistant to push the anterior jugular out of the way, the surgeon applies Kocher clamps across the upper aspects of the prethyroid muscle from the median side toward the lateral side (Fig. 12–6). The prethyroid muscles are then divided between the clamps.

A Lahey double hook clamp is applied over the Kocher clamp for traction on the upper portion of the divided prethyroid muscles. Extreme gentleness is necessary to retract the upper portion of the divided prethyroid muscles to expose the upper pole and the superior thyroid vessels. This is aided by gentle downward traction on the gland. To allow better elevation of the prethyroid muscles and better exposure of the

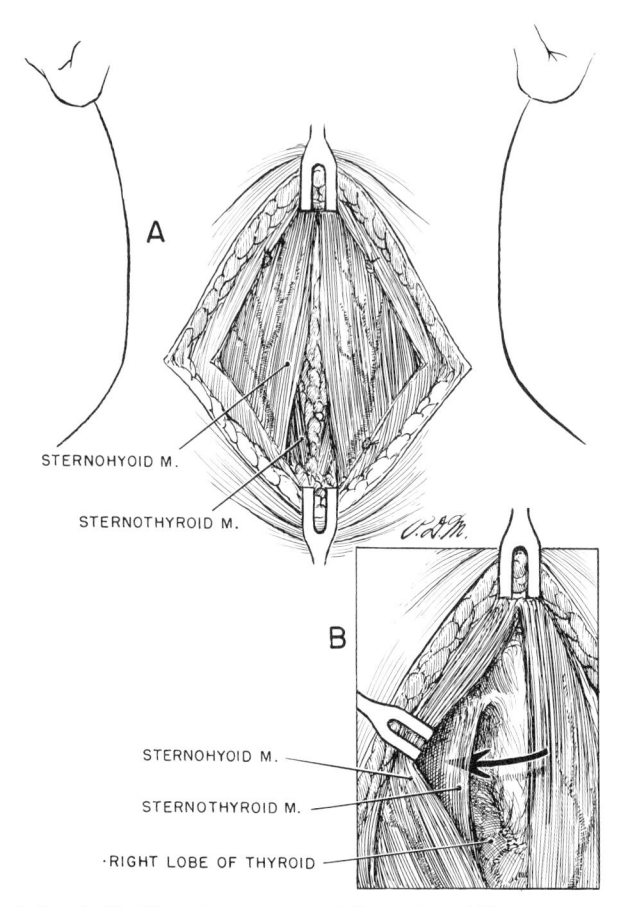

Figure 12-5. *A*, Dividing the pretracheal fascia in midline from below upward. Midline is best identified low in neck. Frequently there is a small amount of fat indicating the site of the midline. *B*, Freeing thyroid capsule from the sternothyroid muscle. Sternohyoid muscle is retracted laterally. Medial border of sternothyroid is identified, and muscle is separated from thyroid capsule. Arrow indicates plane between sternothyroid muscle and thyroid capsule.

superior pole, fibers of the omohyoid joining the lateral border of the prethyroid muscles may be divided. As the area of the superior pole is unroofed, I have found it advantageous to incise the sternothyroid muscle below its attachment to the thyroid cartilage (Fig. 12-7). As the sternothyroid crosses the superior pole to the thyroid cartilage, it prevents further elevation of the sternohyoid and permits access to the superior thyroid vessels. The plane between the sternohyoid and the sternothyroid is avascular. If this plane is entered, the sternothyroid may be divided. The sternohyoid is then further elevated and the superior thyroid vessels are well exposed in the operative field, although covered by a few fibers of the sternothyroid (Fig. 12-7). The lower divided pre-

Surgical Technique

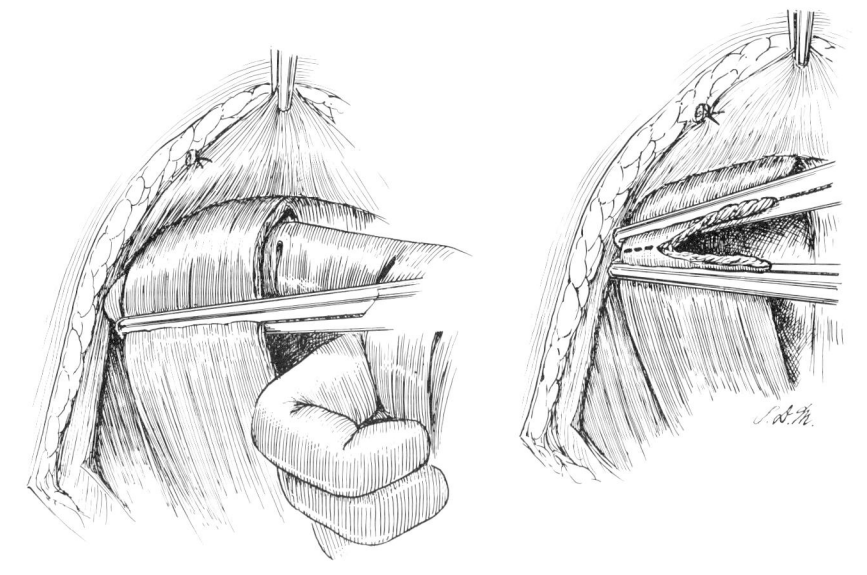

Figure 12-6. Cutting the prethyroid muscles high to avoid injury to the ansa hypoglossi which descends along the lateral border of the muscle, entering the muscle low in the neck.

thyroid muscles are freed laterally and retracted downward. Both lobes are exposed in the same manner and the anterior exposure of the thyroid is completed (Fig. 12–8).

If the anterior exposure has been performed properly, the remainder of the operation should go smoothly. Difficulty encountered

Figure 12-7. Exposure of the superior thyroid pole. The sternothyroid muscle inserts into the thyroid cartilage. The sternohyoid muscle inserts higher in the neck into the hyoid. The sternothyroid muscle fibers are divided, allowing the sternohyoid to be retracted more cephalad to expose the superior pole. The superior thyroid pole is exposed but covered with fibers of sternothyroid.

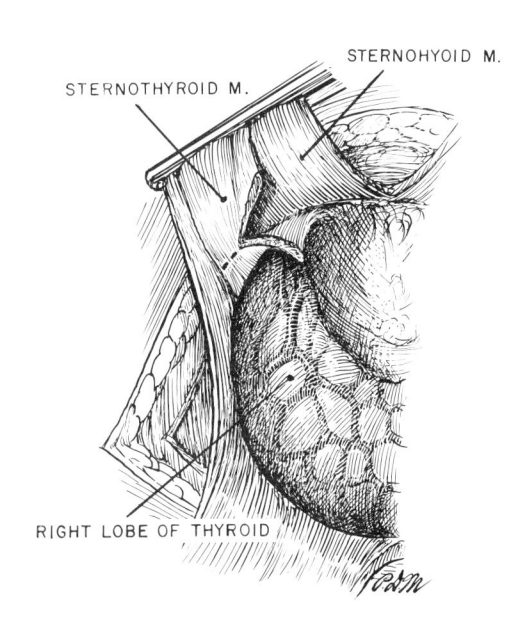

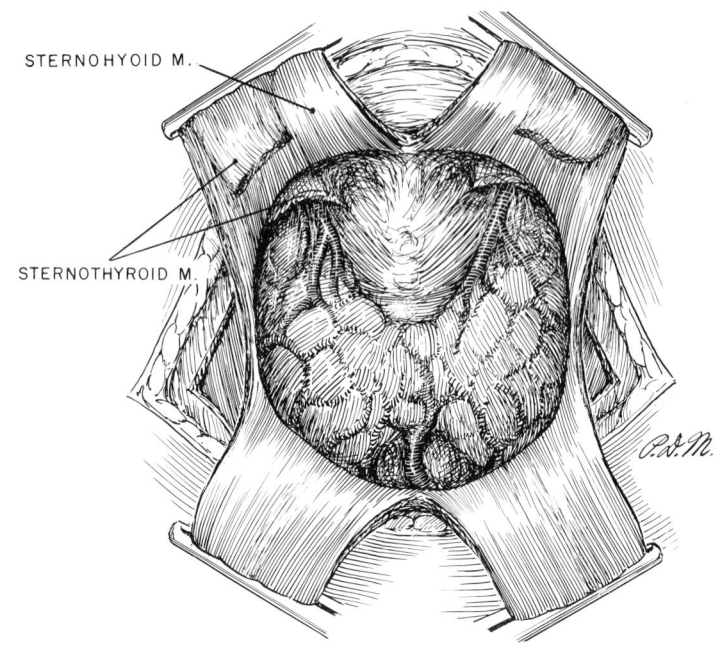

Figure 12–8. Completed anterior exposure.

with mobilization, hemorrhage, and identification of the recurrent nerves and the parathyroids is usually the result of poor anterior exposure.

Mobilization of the Gland

The mobilization of the thyroid gland involves division of the lateral thyroid veins so that the internal jugular vein and carotid artery can be retracted laterally and the thyroid displaced up and out of its bed (Fig. 12–9 *A* and *B*). This gives access to the inferior thyroid aspect of the gland so that the inferior thyroid artery can be isolated and the recurrent laryngeal nerve identified. The numbers of lateral veins are variable. There is usually one vein at the upper pole, two or more veins draining the middle third of the gland, and frequently a plexus of veins in the region of the inferior pole. Gentle upward and medial traction on the gland places the lateral veins on the stretch so that by meticulous dissection they may be clamped and severed. As the lateral veins empty directly into the internal jugular vein, an inadvertent tear may flood the lateral compartment, making later identification of the inferior thyroid artery and recurrent laryngeal nerve more difficult. In large goiters the lateral veins should be divided close to the capsule. If the gland is retracted anteriorly and medially, the cleavage plane will be apparent. An unfortunate accident, which results from rough surgery, is avulsion of a

SURGICAL TECHNIQUE

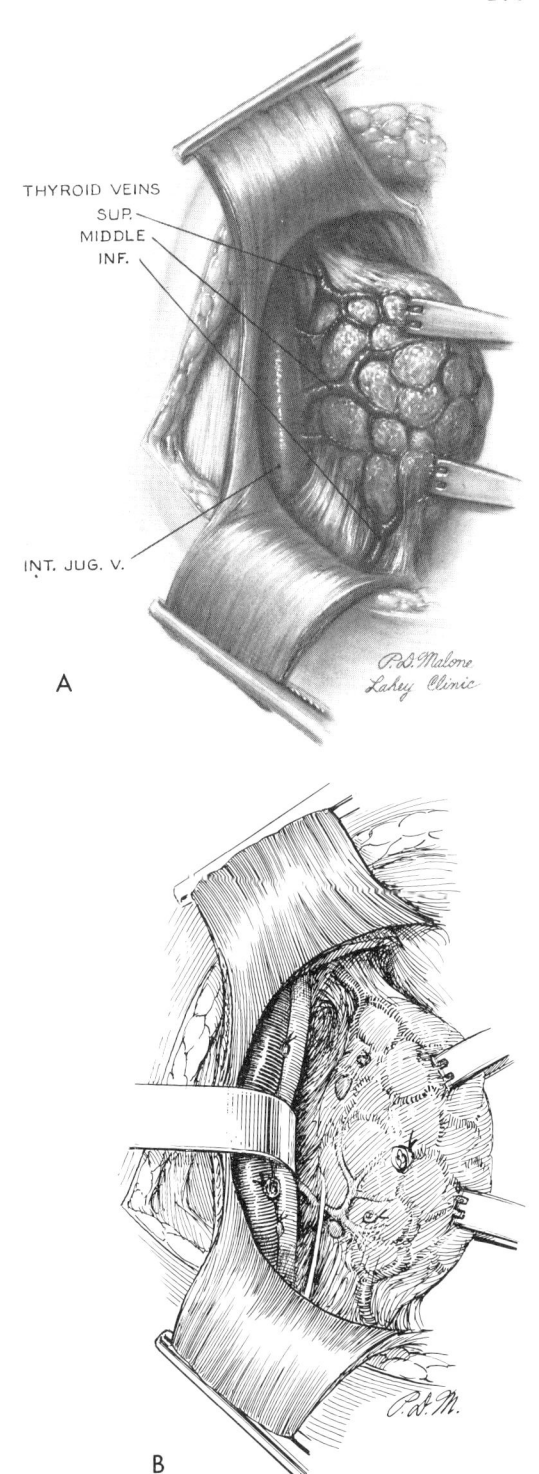

Figure 12-9. A, Exposure of lateral veins. B, The lateral veins have been ligated and divided. The thyroid gland has been lifted up out of its bed. The internal jugular vein and carotid artery are retracted laterally, and the lateral compartment is exposed for visualization of the recurrent laryngeal nerve and inferior thyroid artery.

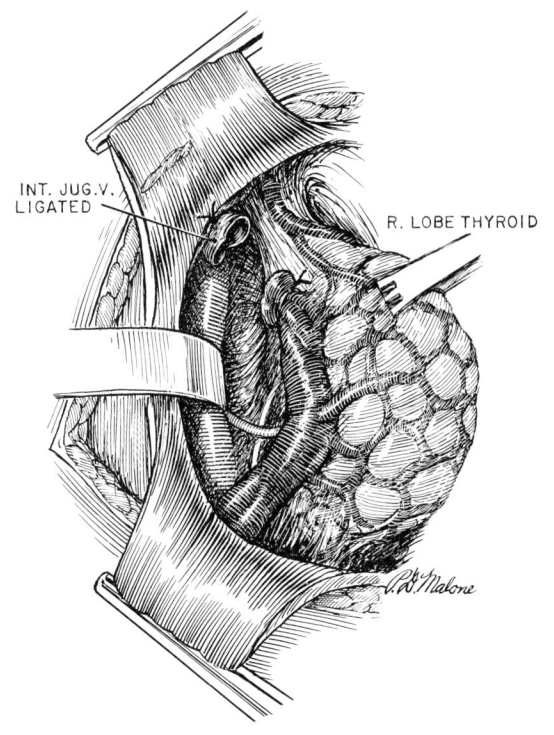

Figure 12–10. Large goiter with internal jugular vein and lateral inferior thyroid veins appearing clearly adherent to thyroid capsule. If these are not recognized, the dissection may occur between the internal jugular vein and carotid artery with inadvertent excision of the internal jugular vein with the gland.

middle thyroid vein, producing a tear in the lateral wall of the internal jugular vein. As mentioned in the chapter on surgical anatomy, in large goiters that have expanded laterally, the cleavage plane between the capsule of the gland and the internal jugular vein may not immediately be apparent. The internal jugular vein may be tightly adherent to the capsule and the lateral veins may be pushed medially onto the capsule (Fig. 12–10). In large goiters the lateral veins should be divided close to the capsule. If the gland is rotated anteriorly and medially, the cleavage plane will be apparent, the internal jugular vein visualized and retracted laterally, and the remaining lateral veins severed. I have known surgeons who misinterpret this situation and inadvertently excise the internal jugular vein and the lateral thyroid veins with the gland.

Isolation of the Inferior Thyroid Artery

The most vulnerable location for injury to the recurrent laryngeal nerve is the point at which the inferior thyroid artery approaches the lateral aspect of the thyroid. Before entering the thyroid gland, the infe-

Surgical Technique

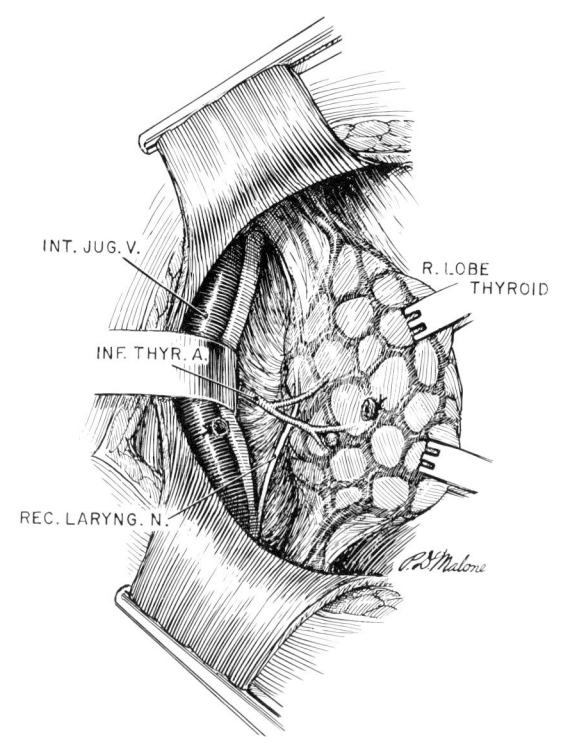

Figure 12-11. Relationship of inferior thyroid artery and recurrent laryngeal nerve.

rior thyroid artery may divide into one or more branches and be intermittently associated with the recurrent laryngeal nerve and its branches (Fig. 12-11). For those not familiar with these all-important anatomical relationships, the reader is referred to the chapter on surgical anatomy. The localization of the internal thyroid artery is important not only for control of bleeding but also because it plays an important part in identification of the recurrent laryngeal nerve.

The internal jugular vein and the carotid artery are retracted laterally and the thyroid gland is retracted anteriorly and medially, exposing the entire posterior lateral edge of the thyroid. It must be emphasized that for easy identification of the inferior thyroid artery and the recurrent laryngeal nerve, this compartment should be free of blood and blood-stained tissues. By meticulous scissors dissection in this avascular field, the inferior thyroid artery will be visualized coming from beneath the carotid artery, in most instances at the level of the midportion of the thyroid gland. Occasionally it appears as high as the superior pole and in such cases, as it descends, it divides in two branches. This division may occur behind the carotid sheath and present what appears to be a double inferior thyroid artery. Infrequently it is found at the level of the inferior pole coming straight upward into the gland. As the inferior thyroid artery is followed to the capsule of the gland, attention is directed to the recurrent laryngeal nerve which, in most cases, passes inferior to the artery but may be above or between the branches of the artery.

To prevent damage to the recurrent laryngeal nerve the inferior thyroid artery is not ligated until the nerve is isolated and out of the way. The artery is then ligated in continuity free of surrounding tissue as far laterally as possible.

Tying the inferior thyroid artery in continuity reduces the risk of a blown-off tie, a serious complication. Although tying the inferior thyroid artery laterally may occlude the branch of the artery supplying the inferior parathyroid, we have not experienced any parathyroid deficiency even though both inferior and superior thyroid arteries on both sides have been ligated.

Hemorrhage from a torn inferior thyroid artery is inexcusable. Obviously it cannot be controlled with pressure on the carotid artery, as is possible with a torn superior thyroid artery. If this catastrophe occurs, the carotid sheath must be retracted laterally and anteriorly and the proximal end of the artery clamped and ligated.

Isolation of the Recurrent Laryngeal Nerve

Before the tie on the inferior thyroid artery is secured, the recurrent laryngeal nerve must be demonstrated. Again, a thorough knowledge of the anatomical relationships of the artery and nerve, adequate exposure, a good light, and an avascular field are of paramount importance. Most often the recurrent nerve is identified at the time the inferior thyroid artery is isolated. If not, it is sought low in the neck in its usual position in the groove between the esophagus and the trachea.

As it approaches the lower border of the thyroid it may, as it ascends, turn as much as 1 cm. lateral to this groove and be intimately associated with a plexus of delicate inferior thyroid veins. Bleeding is avoided by meticulous scissors dissection, always opening the scissors in the direction of the course of the nerve. The recurrent laryngeal nerve may have one or more extralaryngeal branches. Only one, however, contains the motor fibers supplying the laryngeal muscles. From a practical point of view, all branches must be considered as possible motor branches and spared injury. Once identified, the nerve is followed to its junction with the inferior thyroid artery. The inferior thyroid artery is then ligated in continuity.

Mobilization of the Inferior Pole

With the inferior thyroid artery ligated and the recurrent nerve visualized, the lower pole may be mobilized safely. The midline of the

Surgical Technique

Figure 12-12. Ligation of inferior thyroid vessels. Clamps applied from medial to lateral. Recurrent nerve in view and protected. Two clamps are placed below to ensure vessels from inadvertently slipping into mediastinum.

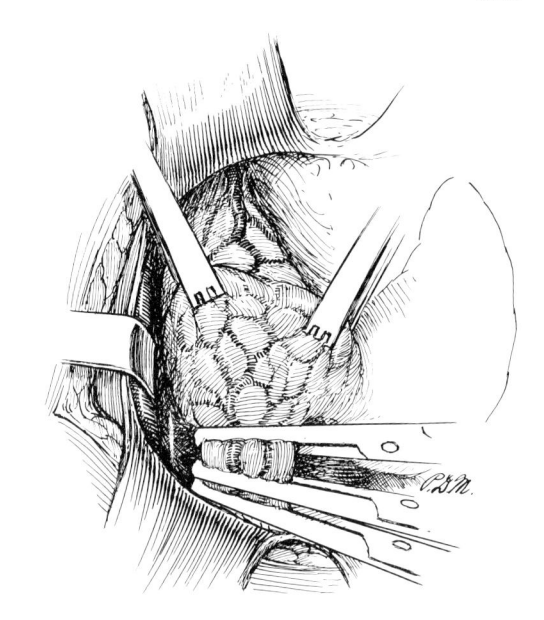

trachea is demonstrated below the isthmus. The entire plexus of vessels below the isthmus and inferior poles (occasionally the thyroidea ima vessels) may be cross-clamped (Fig. 12-12). During this maneuver the recurrent nerve is constantly in view. The clamps are applied from the midline out. We prefer to use two hemostats below and one above and divide between the upper one and the lower two. This is a safety measure and prevents any possibility of the vessels slipping from one clamp and escaping into the mediastinum, where they may be difficult to retrieve. With the vessel divided, the lower pole is gently detached from the trachea and pulled upward.

Division of the Superior Thyroid Vessels and Mobilization of the Upper Pole

The superior thyroid vessels must be ligated under direct vision. With high elevation of the prethyroid muscle and downward and inward traction of the superior pole, they can be separated from the inferior constrictor muscle. They may be hidden beneath a few fibers of the divided sternothyroid. It is best to ligate the vessels with a ligature passing from inside out. The vessels are doubly ligated above and divided between the ligatures and a clamp placed below (Fig. 12-13). As previously described (Chapter 3, Surgical Anatomy), these vessels may approach the upper pole of the thyroid along its anterior and inner aspect. In hyperplastic glands a lingula or tongue of the thyroid tissue may ascend

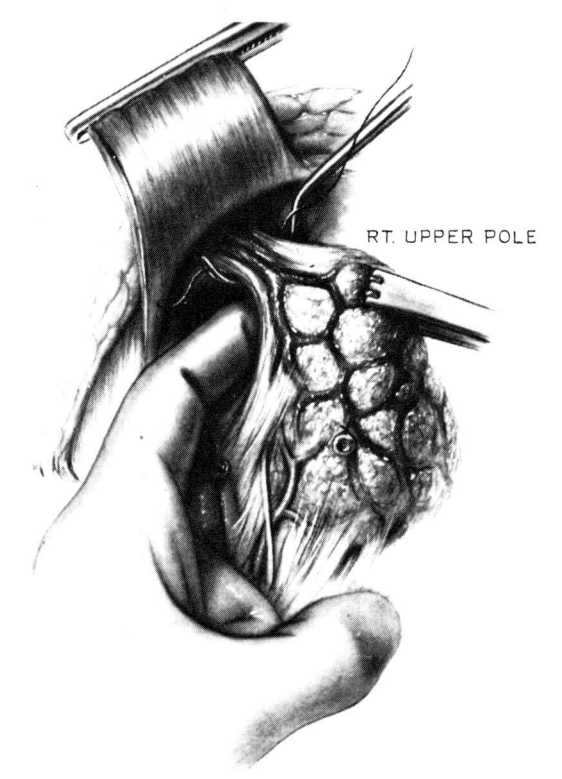

Figure 12-13. Ligation of superior polar vessels. These are doubly ligated and divided.

Surgical Technique

high lateral to the entry of the vessels into the gland. In such instances two mistakes may be made:

1. A blind attempt may be made to pass a ligature around the vessels above the lingula.

2. The lingula may be transected with the vessels, leaving remaining thyroid tissue intact, a possible and frequent focus for recurrence in Graves' disease and a difficult problem to excise at a later date. This may be avoided by isolating and dividing the superior thyroid vessels at a lower level and then, by excising the thyroid capsule, this extension of thyroid tissue made by inward and downward traction may be enucleated. Before complete enucleation, small posterior veins entering the gland should be clamped (Fig. 12-14).

Identification of the Parathyroids

At this stage of thyroidectomy, with full exposure now obtained, the parathyroids should be identified. Every attempt is made to preserve at least one parathyroid on each side. Their locations are amazingly constant and, with experience, they are easy to find. As familiarity is gained with their appearance—pea-size, lima bean-shaped, molded edges, mahogany brown in color, appearing as distinct organs close to the thyroid capsule—they become more readily identified. Operative trauma or bruising of the parathyroids or adjacent lymph nodes may result in some capsular hemorrhage, staining the tissues so that the thyroid, parathyroid fat, and lymphatic tissues are not clearly differentiated.

Once the superior pole is rotated downward and inward, the superior parathyroid may be seen at about the junction of the upper and

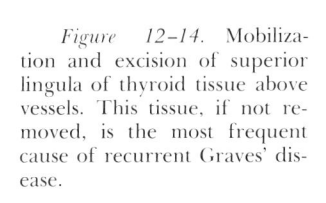

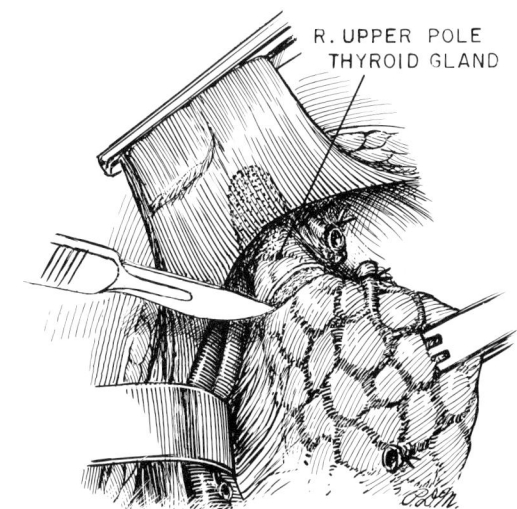

Figure 12-14. Mobilization and excision of superior lingula of thyroid tissue above vessels. This tissue, if not removed, is the most frequent cause of recurrent Graves' disease.

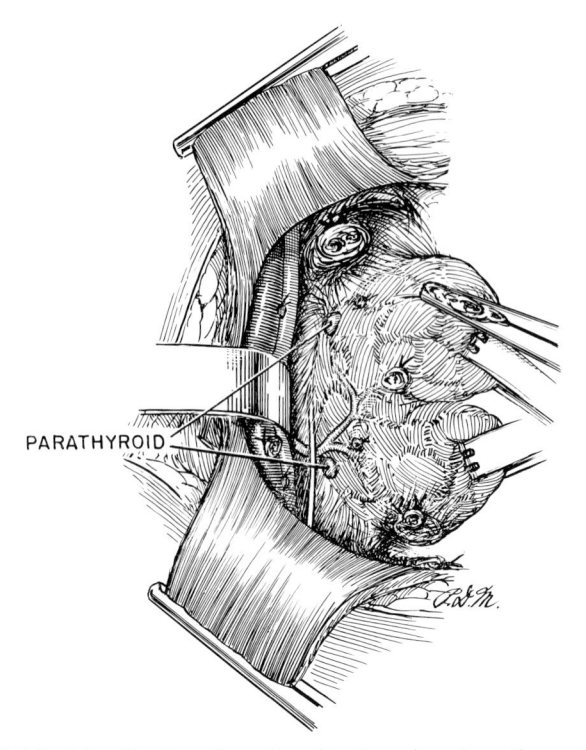

Figure 12-15. Identification of parathyroids. Superior, along the posterior capsule about the junction of the upper and middle thirds of the gland. Inferior, at the junction of the inferior thyroid artery and recurrent laryngeal nerve.

middle thirds of thyroid glands along its lateral posterior aspect (Fig. 12-15). The inferior parathyroids are usually found close to the junction of the inferior thyroid artery and the recurrent laryngeal nerves. Frequently a branch of the inferior thyroid artery leads to the inferior parathyroid. Clamps should be inserted into the thyroid capsule anterior to the parathyroids, and the capsule and the parathyroids gently dislodged from the thyroid gland so that they are not excised with the resected gland.

Division of the Isthmus

The isthmus is freed from its attachment to the trachea in the midline from below upward by blunt dissection and divided between a series of hemostats (Fig.12-16). Care must be exercised in separating the isthmus from the underlying pretracheal fascia to avoid puncture of the trachea by the sharp points of this straight clamp. At the upper aspect of the isthmus the suspensory ligament is divided to complete the mobilization of the gland. A series of clamps is placed along the medial capsule

Surgical Technique

and the capsule is incised above the clamps, producing a cuff, outlining the medial border of the resection.

At this moment in thyroidectomy it is necessary to determine the amount of gland to resect or, conversely, the amount of gland to be left. This is determined by the pathologic condition for which thyroidectomy is being performed. In hyperthyroidism it may depend upon the severity of the thyrotoxicosis and the age of the patient. Usually about 90 percent of the gland should be removed, or 1 to 2 gm. left behind. With a diffuse hyperplastic gland such as is found in Graves' disease, it is better to err on the side of more radical removal, as surgically produced hypothyroidism is more easily controlled than recurrent hyperthyroidism. In toxic nodular goiters the incidence of postoperative hypothyroidism is almost zero, and the size of the remaining remnant is not so critical. In the nontoxic nodular goiter, a larger remnant may be left so that the patient's preoperative thyroid requirements may be met without additional thyroid supplement, although at times suppressive therapy may be necessary to control recurrence of the goiter. In chronic thyroiditis, removal of the gland may be necessary for relief of discomfort or pressure symptoms. The majority of patients with chronic thyroiditis will have myxedema, or it will develop regardless of the amount of gland removed. In benign tumors less radical subtotal lobectomy to remove the

Figure 12–16. Division of the isthmus and incision of medial capsule. Incision of lateral capsules and excision of thyroid gland. If total thyroidectomy is to be performed, the recurrent nerve is followed to its entrance into the larynx.

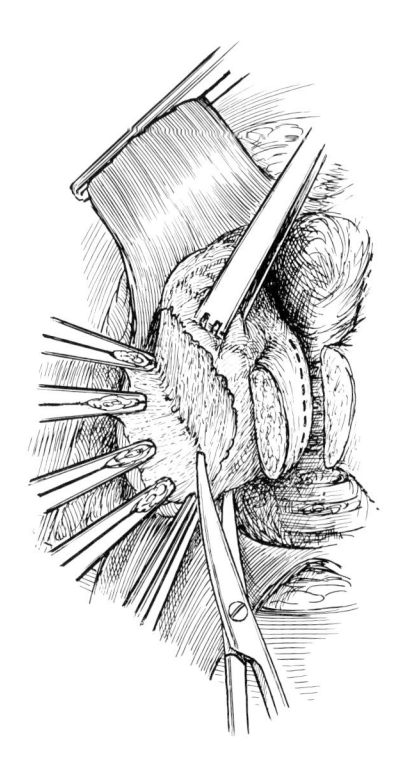

tumor completely will suffice. In malignant tumors total thyroidectomy may be indicated. Judgment as to the size of a remnant to be left comes with experience.

The recurrent laryngeal nerve and the parathyroids are again visualized to prevent injury. With the superior and inferior poles mobilized and the gland retracted medially, hemostats are applied to the lateral capsule, outlining the amount of thyroid to be removed (Fig. 12–16). The capsule is incised above the line of hemostats. The thyroid tissue will appear to bulge out of the capsule. The incised lower edge of the capsule is pushed downward to help to preserve the parathyroids and their blood supply. A cuff of thyroid capsule and thyroid tissue is developed which will clearly establish the lateral border of the remnant and will later be sutured to the medial cuff to reconstruct the remnant.

The thyroid tissue between the lateral and medial lines of hemostats now outlines the boundaries of the thyroid to be excised. By the clamp and cut technique within the thyroid capsule, the gland is excised to free it from the remaining remnant (Fig. 12–16). All vessels are tied and hemostasis is assured. The remnant is reconstructed by suturing the lateral thyroid capsule to the medial capsule. If the medial capsule is not well defined, the sutures may be placed in the pretracheal fascia to buttress the cut edge of the gland against the trachea. To avoid injury to the recurrent laryngeal nerve, sutures should not be placed deep in the tissue of the remnant (Fig. 12–17 *A*).

The left subtotal hemithyroidectomy is performed in exactly the same manner. It should be noted that a pyramidal lobe, if present, is more common on the left; it may be small and consequently overlooked. Recurrent hyperthyroidism following thyroidectomy for Graves' disease most often develops secondary to thyroid tissue left either at the superior poles or as an overlooked pyramidal lobe. Even though an overlooked pyramidal lobe is small in a patient with Graves' disease, it may become hyperplastic after thyroidectomy and produce signs and symptoms of hyperplasia, and the patient will return with a sausage-like mass in the front of the neck. This may be avoided by carefully looking for the pyramidal lobe and excising it completely up to the hyoid (Fig. 12–17 *B*).

CLOSURE OF THE WOUND

The head is slightly flexed to remove tension on the prethyroid muscles. The prethyroid muscles are approximated with mattress sutures (Fig. 12–17 *C*). The anterior jugular vein, if unusually large, should be ligated separately. I have seen instances in which these vessels retract from the mattress sutures approximating the prethyroid muscles and cause postoperative hemorrhage. We do not suture the platysma. The skin edges are approximated with skin clips (Fig. 12–17 *D*). The excellence of the scar depends upon careful approximation of the skin

SURGICAL TECHNIQUE 189

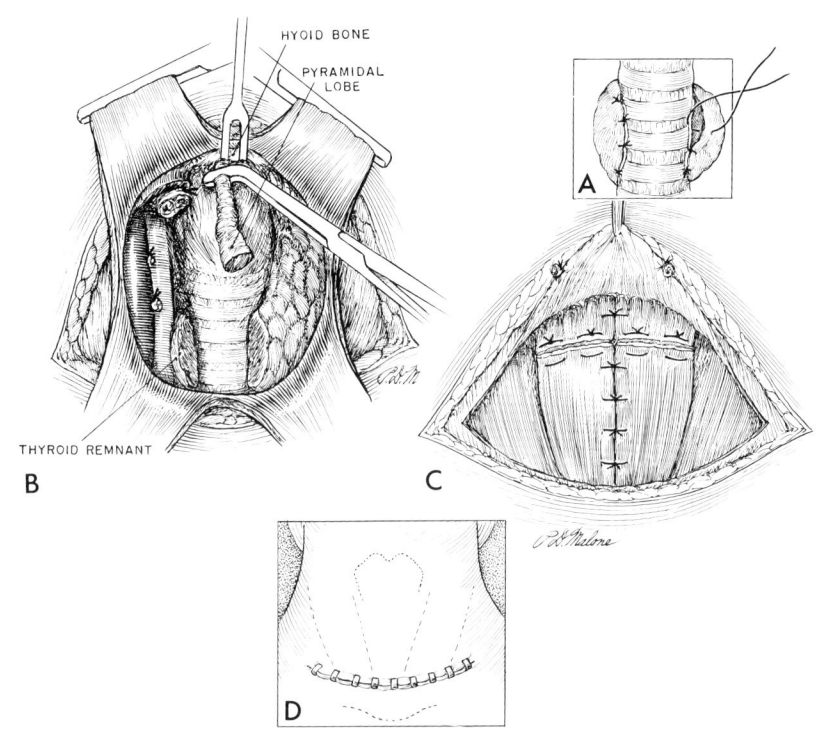

Figure 12-17. *A,* Reconstruction of thyroid remnant. The lateral thyroid capsule is sutured to the medial thyroid capsule or pretracheal fascia. *B,* Excision of pyramidal lobe. It usually arises from the left side and should be excised up to the hyoid. If not removed in hyperplastic glands, it may produce recurrent Graves' disease. *C,* Closure of muscles. *D,* Closure with skin clips.

edges. Ordinarily drains are not necessary; if they are used, they are brought out at the angles of the incision. Half of the clips are taken out on the second postoperative day and the remainder on the third postoperative day.

THYROIDECTOMY COMBINED WITH NECK DISSECTION

The indicated surgical procedure for malignant disease of the thyroid is discussed elsewhere. The operative techniques involved are total lobectomy on the side involved and radical subtotal thyroidectomy on the opposite side, or thyroidectomy combined with a modified or complete radical neck dissection. Total thyroidectomy is performed with few exceptions by the same technical steps described for subtotal thyroidectomy. Defining the lateral and medial borders of the remnant is eliminated. After complete mobilization of the lateral aspects of the gland, the poles, and the isthmus, the inferior thyroid artery is ligated and the recurrent laryngeal nerve is dissected free of all tissue to its entry into the larynx. The gland is then excised completely from its bed, leaving the trachea bare of all thyroid tissue.

The diagnosis of malignant disease may be confirmed before radical neck dissection either by previous cervical lymph node biopsy or excisional thyroid biopsy; or the diagnosis may be made by frozen section at the time of thyroidectomy. In most cases, particularly in women with thin necks, the limb of the collar incision may be extended laterally (horseshoe type), the skin flaps further elevated, and satisfactory exposure obtained (Fig. 12-18 B). In obese patients and those with lateral scars from previous biopsy of cervical nodes, a long incision is made extending from the mastoid process along the anterior medial border of the sternocleidomastoid muscle to the suprasternal notch. The incision is then carried above the clavicle backward to the trapezius muscle (Fig. 12-18 A). Regardless of the type of incision, skin flaps must be raised to expose the superficial structures of the neck from the sternum and clavicle below, the area of the parotid and thyroid cartilage above, the entire thyroid lobe of the opposite side, and the anterior border of the trapezius behind the gland (Fig. 12-19). The sternothyroid, sternohyoid, and sternocleidomastoid are divided from their attachments to the sternum and clavicle.

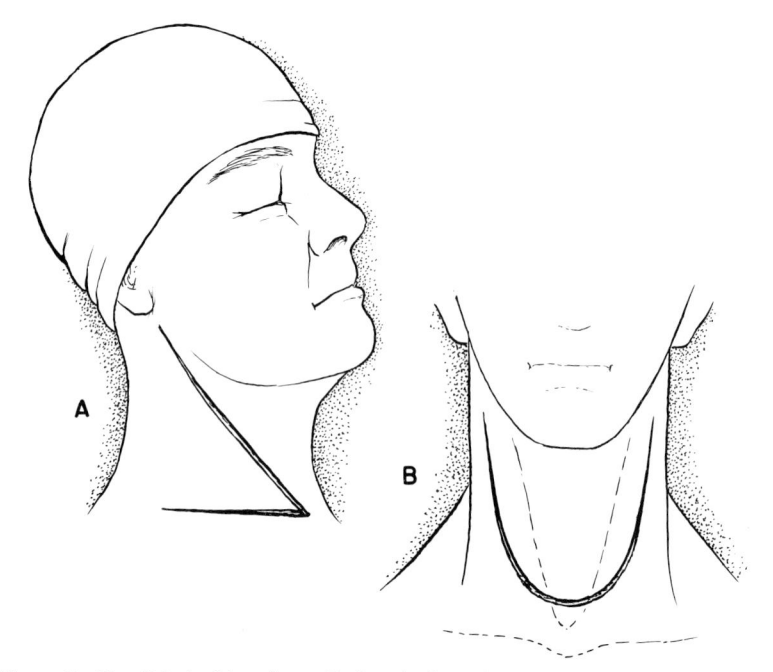

Figure 12-18. Skin incision for radical neck dissection. *A*, Classic, and *B*, horseshoe.

Surgical Technique

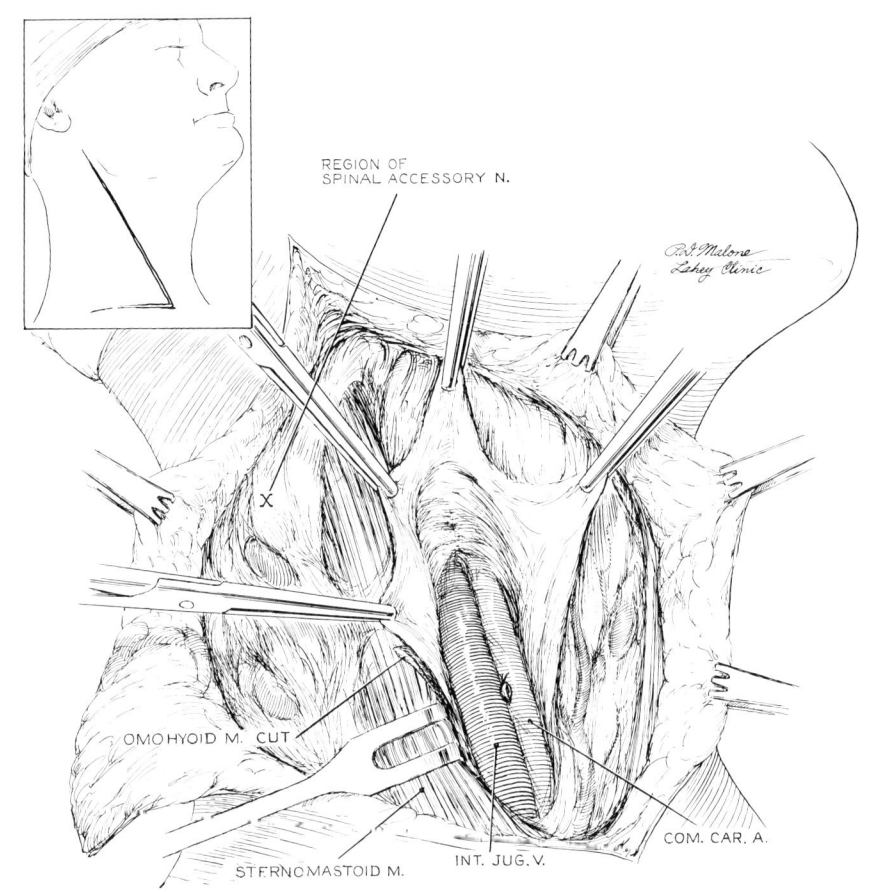

Figure 12-19. Anterior exposure for radical neck dissection. Wide exposure made possible by dissection between skin flap and lateral retraction. X — region of spinal accessory nerve. Note complete separation of the internal jugular vein and the common carotid artery in front of the sternocleidomastoid to make early ligation of the internal jugular vein at its lowest possible point.

The inferior thyroid veins (the thyroidea ima vessels when present) are divided in the midline. The internal jugular vein is isolated from its attachment to the carotid sheath. At this level the vagus nerve is identified between the internal jugular vein and the carotid artery. The internal jugular vein is divided low in the neck and the entire mass of lymphatics, muscles, and veins is retracted upward and dissected en bloc away from the underlying muscles and deeper structures, including the brachial plexus (Fig. 12-20). As the dissection proceeds upward in this avascular plane afforded by the carotid sheath, the phrenic and spinal accessory nerves are identified to avoid injury. If a total thyroidectomy has not been previously performed, as the dissection approaches the lower pole of the thyroid the isthmus is freed, the inferior thyroid artery

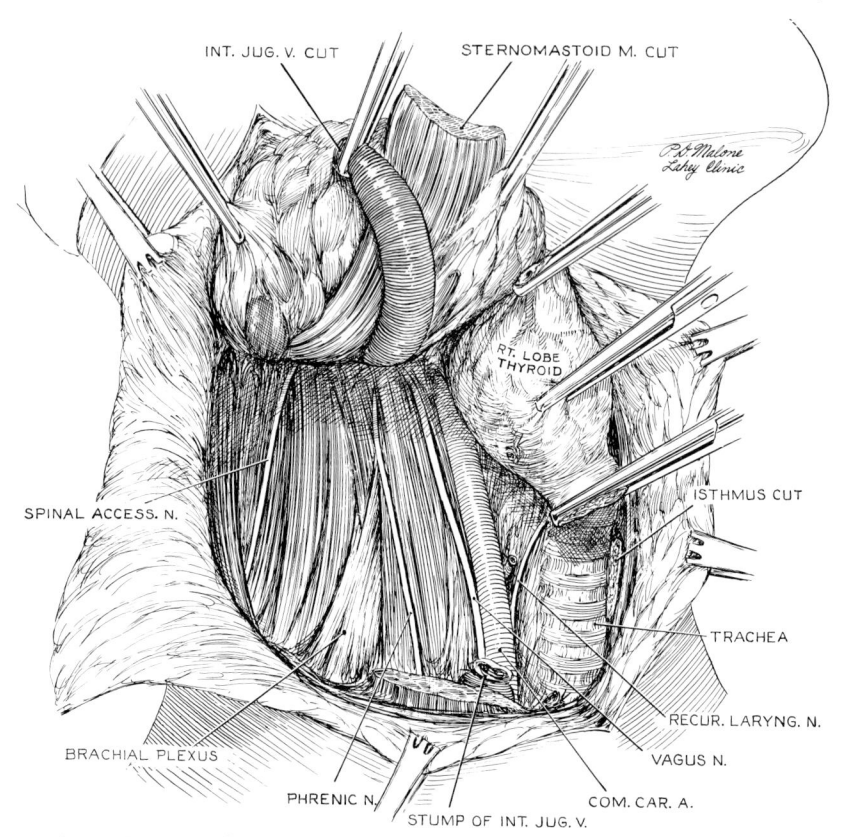

Figure 12–20. Radical neck dissection. The sternocleidomastoid muscle has been severed, the internal jugular vein ligated and divided, and the dissection performed along the carotid sheath from below upward, exposing the underlying structures. The thyroid gland is dissected free from the trachea, sparing the recurrent laryngeal nerve.

is ligated, the course of the recurrent laryngeal nerve is followed to the larynx, and the remaining thyroid gland is excised from the trachea. The dissection is completed by excision of the insertion of the prethyroid muscles, high ligation of the internal jugular vein, and severance of the sternocleidomastoid at the level of the parotid gland (Fig. 12–21).

FREEING A SUBSTERNAL GOITER

In our experience, almost all substernal goiters may be removed through the neck. On most occasions venous hemorrhage is more troublesome than arterial hemorrhage. Venous hemorrhage before delivery of a substernal goiter into the neck may be serious. The superficial and deep thyroid veins may be greatly enlarged and dilated secondary to the tourniquet effect of the goiter pressing on the superior thoracic strait. Extreme care must be exercised to avoid tearing these veins. If serious

SURGICAL TECHNIQUE 193

venous bleeding does occur, the substernal goiter must be rapidly delivered from the superior mediastinum. The tourniquet effect is then released, the veins will collapse, and hemorrhage is controlled. It is to be remembered that the arterial supply to the substernal goiter arises in the neck, and it should be ligated, if possible, before attempting the enucleation. After ligation of the inferior thyroid and superior thyroid arteries, a cleavage plane is sought between the capsule of the thyroid and the surrounding tissue. The trachea may be compressed and pushed to one side. The best cleavage plane is usually laterally and posteriorly. By finger dissection the goiter is freed from the pleura and cellular tissue in the mediastinum and is delivered into the neck (Fig. 12-22). If the tumor is not carcinomatous and the substernal goiter cannot be freed by enucleation, the method described by Dr. Lahey may be useful (Fig. 12-22): The capsule of the goiter is opened and its contents which are usually seminecrotic or semicystic, are broken down and scooped out,

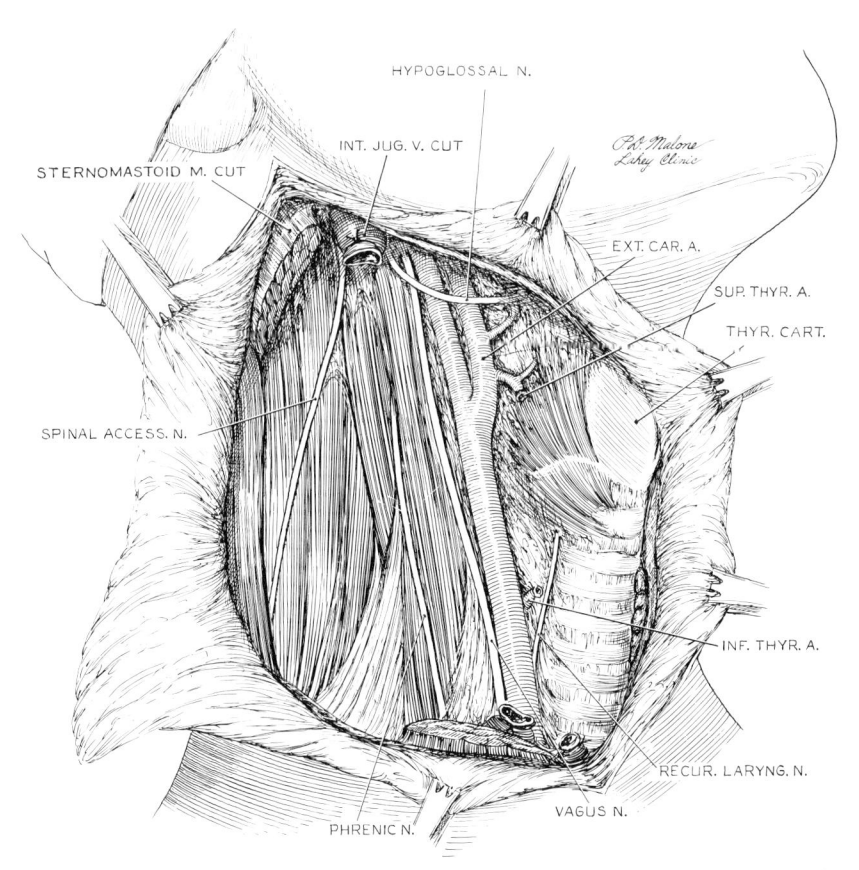

Figure 12-21. Radical neck dissection completed. The internal jugular vein is ligated below and above. The spinal accessory, recurrent laryngeal, and vagus nerves are intact. Small remnant of thyroid gland remains on opposite side.

thus decreasing its diameter. Then with gentle, gradual traction upward, with finger dissection outside the capsule to free it from the pleura, it may be delivered without further difficulty. It is only rarely that a transsternal approach is necessary for such goiters.

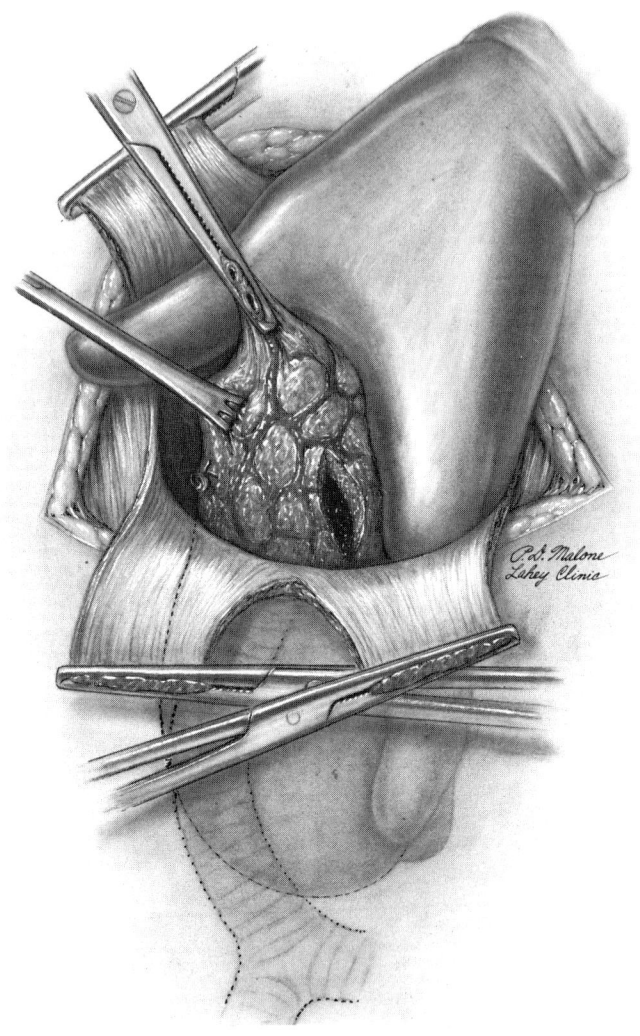

Figure 12–22. Finger dissection of substernal goiter. Note that the index finger is inserted into the mediastinum outside the thyroid capsule and is swept around until the gland is freed from the pleura and cellular tissue in the mediastinum. This may be the first step in removing intrathyroid goiter so as to release the tourniquet effect of the clavicles on the thyroid veins and to reduce hemorrhage. Occasionally the substernal goiter cannot be made to pass out of the superior thoracic strait. In such cases, if one encounters venous hemorrhage from the tourniquet effect at the superior thoracic outlet, it may be necessary to enter the thyroid capsule and scoop out the contents, thus decreasing its diameter and reducing hemorrhage. Then, with gentle upward traction on the capsule, the gland is further separated with the index finger outside the capsule, freeing it from the pleura and surrounding structures.

SURGICAL TECHNIQUE 195

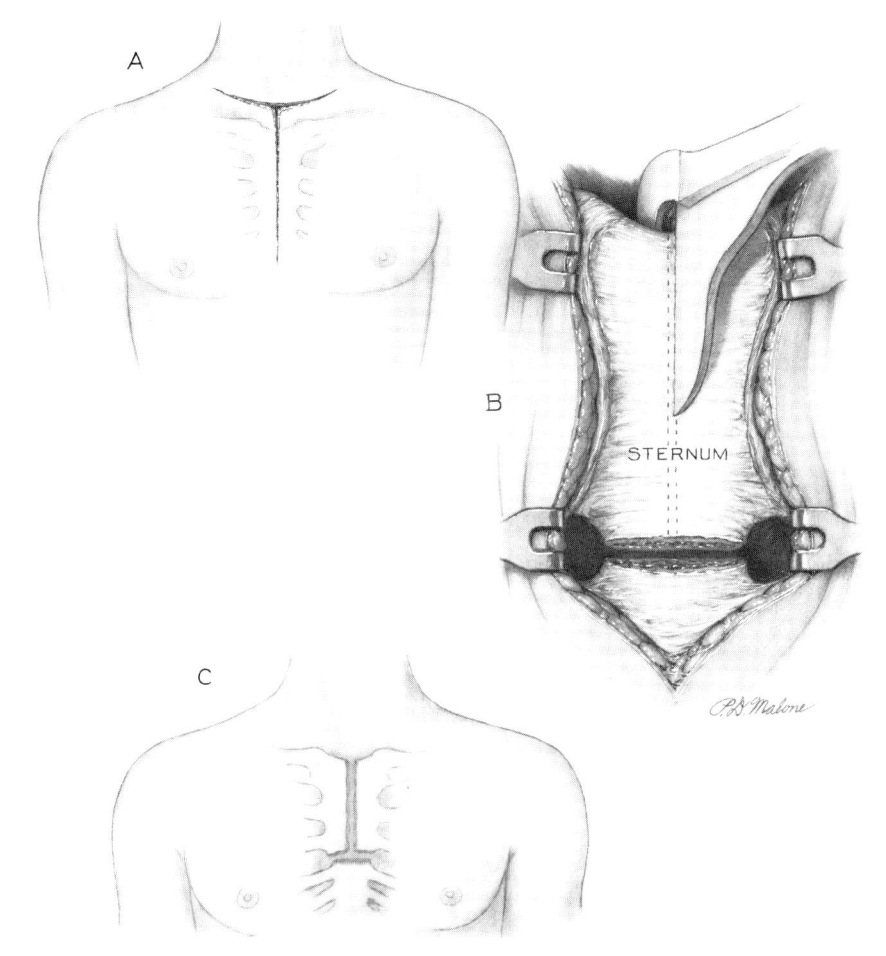

Figure 12–23. Technique of cervicomediastinotomy.

TRANSSTERNAL MEDIASTINOTOMY

The thyroid surgeon should be familiar with a method to expose the anterior-superior mediastinum. This may be necessary to remove a large substernal goiter or to perform anterior-superior mediastinal dissection for malignant disease.

A vertical incision is made from the midportion of the collar incision at the substernal notch in the midline downward to the level of the border of the fourth costal cartilage (Fig. 12–23). The sternum is bared down to the periosteum. The intercostal muscles in the third interspace close to the sternum are divided and separated on each side. The undersurface of the sternum is freed by blunt dissection and divided transversely at this level. Using a sternal cutter, the manubrium and upper

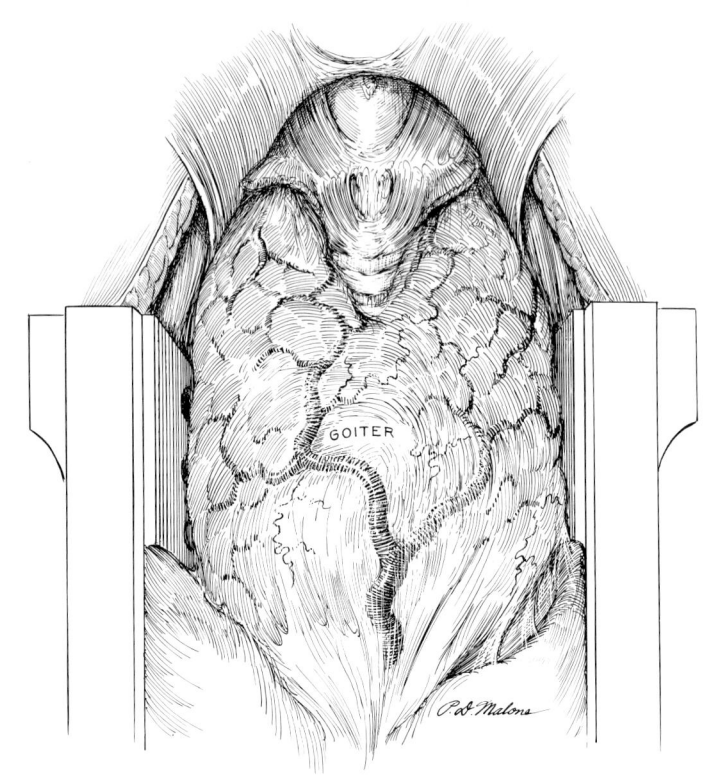

Figure 12-24. Exposure of intrathoracic goiter obtained by cervicomediastinotomy.

sternum are cut vertically in the midline down to the transected sternum. Mediastinal tissues are further dissected from the undersurface of the sternum and the attached cartilages. The divided sternum is retracted laterally and wide exposure to the anterior surface of the mediastinum is obtained (Fig. 12-24). Beginning at the pericardium, the fascia with the lymph nodes, fibroareolar tissue, thymus, and remaining thyroid remnants are dissected from below upward off the great vessels and the trachea. The recurrent laryngeal nerves are constantly in view (Fig. 12-25). In this fashion the transsternal dissection can be combined with thyroidectomy and radical neck dissection. Closure of the sternum is accomplished by sutures passing through drill holes in the sternum (Fig. 12-26).

THE INTRATHORACIC GOITER

Completely intrathoracic goiters are exceedingly rare, but when they do occur, they may reach considerable size — up to 1,000 gm. They

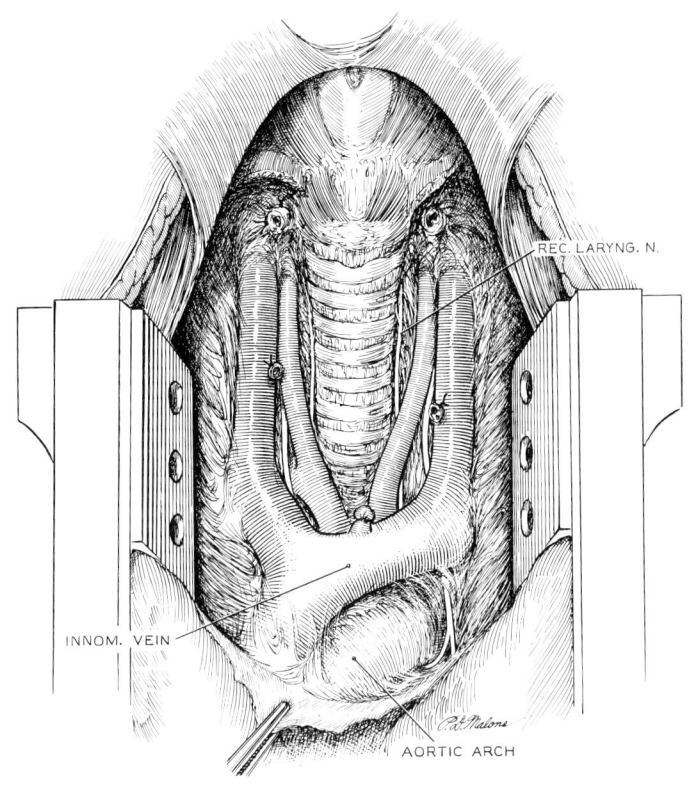

Figure 12–25. Anatomic relationship after removal of intrathoracic goiter and total thyroidectomy.

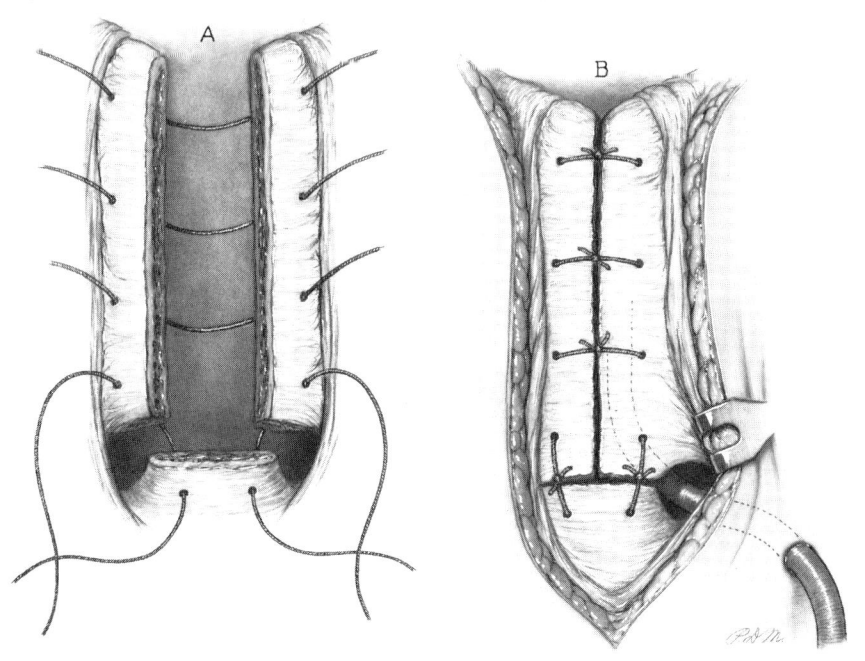

Figure 12–26. Approximation of sternum and closure of the mediastinotomy wound.

197

are intimately associated with the pleura and great vessels and are impossible to remove except through a transthoracic incision. The transpleural approach is used through the right thorax, resecting the sixth rib. A detailed description of transthoracic excision of such intrathoracic lesions is not in the scope of this text, and the reader is referred to texts on thoracic surgery.

POSTOPERATIVE COMPLICATIONS

Postoperative complications may be insignificant, such as edema of the flap, or dangerous and life-threatening, such as hemorrhage or respiratory obstructions. Today, fortunately, because of better preoperative preparation, postoperative complications are few. Most are preventable. The proper management of the patient with thyroid disorder and the surgical technique of thyroidectomy as described previously will keep complications at a minimum. With proper preoperative management, the patient will be euthyroid at the time of surgery. If the patient is hyperthyroid, thyroid storm may occur; if hypothyroid, laryngeal edema may result, producing respiratory obstruction. Careless technique may result in massive hemorrhage, recurrent nerve paralysis, or both, causing respiratory embarrassment. Lack of experience or attention to technical details may involve removal of too little or too much thyroid tissue or possibly all parathyroids, resulting in myxedema, recurrent hyperthyroidism, or parathyroid deficiency. Postoperative complications are related to the wound, hemorrhage, respiratory difficulties, nerve paralysis, recurrent hyperthyroidism or myxedema, or parathyroid deficiency.

Wound Complications

Wound complications include edema of the flap, accumulation of serum, hematoma, or infection. Edema of the flap is secondary to trauma, absorbable sutures, and division of the prethyroid muscles. It occurs more often following thyroidectomy for chronic thyroiditis. It is treated by application of hot, moist soaks. Serum accumulation or hematoma usually occurs on the fourth or fifth day after operation and is evident by fluctuant swelling. It may be kept to a minimum by pressure dressings and may be relieved by aspiration or probing. Frank infection is unusual except when associated with tracheotomy. Heat, drainage, and antibiotics are indicated.

Hemorrhage

Hemorrhage may be of two types: immediate, or delayed. Immediate hemorrhage is the more serious and must be recognized early. It frequently occurs during the postanesthetic period and at the time the endotracheal tube is removed. Its origin may be arterial, or venous from a tear in a large vein. The patient may cough or vomit, producing increased venous pressure, which allows insecure ligatures to dislodge or insignificant vessels to bleed profusely. The surgeon or his assistant must remain with the patient until the endotracheal tube is removed and the patient is breathing quietly.

Profuse hemorrhage may also occur several hours after surgery. It becomes apparent by rapid swelling of the neck and stridor. Blood accumulates beneath the prethyroid muscles, producing pressure on the trachea with subsequent respiratory obstruction. The wound must be opened immediately to release the blood and to allow adequate respiratory exchange. Hemorrhage may be controlled with pressure. An endotracheal tube should be inserted and the patient returned to the operating room. With the patient under anesthesia, the wound is carefully explored, irrigated, and hemostasis assured. If considerable edema is present, tracheostomy should also be performed. Delayed bleeding may occur two or three days after operation and is usually the result of oozing from small veins. The patient's neck will appear swollen and he may complain of tightness in the neck. Usually there is no evidence of respiratory difficulty. Serum and whole blood may be evacuated through an opening in the incision at its lateral aspects.

Respiratory Obstruction

Respiratory obstruction may result from hemorrhage as described above and also from edema of the larynx and vocal cord paralysis. Edema of larynx, vocal cords, and uvula producing an inadequate airway is most common in patients with hypothyroidism, particularly secondary to chronic thyroiditis, or in patients who have been overprepared with antithyroid drugs. A clue to this possibility may be seen by the anesthesiologist at the time of intubation. It must be emphasized that the margin of safety allowing an adequate airway is not great. The patient may have an adequate exchange with a relatively small aperture between the edematous vocal cords. A very slight increase of edema may produce sudden obstruction. A tracheostomy must be performed at the slightest indication of respiratory embarrassment. On occasion a patient will be anxious and nervous, and complain of difficulty in breathing with no evidence of stridor. Steam inhalation and sedation may be all that is necessary. A thyrocardiac will not tolerate any degree of respiratory embarrassment. In such cases a prophylactic tracheostomy should seriously be considered.

Paralysis of one vocal cord may go unnoticed in the postoperative period. However, a paralyzed cord associated with edema may cause stridor and require tracheostomy. Paralysis of both cords will be evident and will be determined at the time of extubation. Paralysis of the cricothyroid muscle by injury to the superior laryngeal nerve is manifested by voice change, weakness, and fatigue. The patient will not be able to reach high notes. Postoperative position of the paralyzed cords is described in the section on anatomy.

Postoperative Hypothyroidism and Hyperthyroidism

The amount of thyroid gland to be left as the remnant has been described in the preceding section on surgical technique of thyroidectomy. Hypothyroidism usually follows surgery for chronic thyroiditis or malignancy. In toxic diffuse glands an error should be made on the side of too little rather than too much. In toxic nodular goiter hypothyroidism is unusual. Preoperative hypothyroidism is controlled by administration of thyroid extract, 2 to 3 grains daily.

Post-thyroidectomy Hypoparathyroidism

Postoperative hypoparathyroidism occurs more frequently after thyroidectomy for Graves' disease or carcinoma. It is manifested by tetany, numbness and tingling of the extremities, and carpopedal spasm. A positive Chvostek's or Trousseau's sign may be elicited. A blood calcium determination confirms the diagnosis. The incidence of permanent hypoparathyroidism at the Lahey Clinic is less than 0.2 percent. Temporary hypoparathyroidism is not serious. It usually is secondary to trauma, that is, pinching, bruising, and so forth, of the parathyroids during the surgical procedure. Temporary hypoparathyroidism may last a few days but may require therapy for several weeks. Tetany may respond initially to 10 to 20 ml. of 10 percent calcium gluconate given intravenously and then require calcium lactate powder orally for several days before the blood calcium is maintained at a normal level.

Permanent hypoparathyroidism is a serious complication. Chronic hypoparathyroidism can result in cataracts, even in the absence of tetany. In patients who have had thyroidectomy, it may be difficult to determine whether the hypoparathyroidism is temporary or permanent, particularly in the few weeks following operation. Any one of the following six signs suggests that a permanent state of hypoparathyroidism may ensue: (1) a triad of positive Chvostek's sign, positive Trousseau's sign, and episodes of convulsions; (2) a low calcium level below 4 mg. per 100 ml. in the postoperative period; (3) an early stable requirement of calcium of over 7 gm. of calcium lactate powder per day; (4) the necessity for adjustment of calcium requirements because stability and a tetany-free state were not obtained during the first 10 days after operation; (5) difficulties in the first few months after operation, so that the patient was unable to work owing to persistent tetany despite frequent medical adjustments; and (6) episodes of neurological disturbances resulting from increased intracranial pressure.*

The aim of medical treatment of hypoparathyroidism is to restore normal blood concentrations of calcium and phosphorus. The adequacy of calcium replacement therapy is gauged by serial determinations of blood calcium. Calcium is given by mouth in the form of calcium lactate powder. Its solubility is increased by giving it in hot fluids. If normal blood calcium levels cannot be established with calcium alone, we add vitamin D_2. Parathyroid hormone is of little help.

---

*Watkins, E., Jr., Bell, G. O., Snow, J. C., and Adams, H. D.: Incidence and current management of post-thyroidectomy hypoparathyroidism. J.A.M.A. *182*:140–146 (Oct. 13) 1962.

Index

Page numbers set in *italics* indicate an illustration.

Achilles stretch reflex test, 63
Adenoma(s) of thyroid gland, 107
   follicular, 37, *37*, *38*
      complications of, 39
Adolescents, antithyroid treatment in, 113
Albucasis, 1
Anesthesia, for emergency surgery for hyperthyroidism, 166
   for surgery of thyroid gland, 153–169
      selection of, 158
Antithyroid drugs, thyroid surgery and, 155
Artery(ies), thyroid, inferior, 15
      isolation of, 180, *181*
      laryngeal nerve and, *19*
      superior, 14
   thyroidea ima, 15
Astwood, 4

Basal metabolic rate, 63
Basedow's disease, 31
Billroth, 2
Bone, carcinoma of, metastatic, 78
Bruberger, 2
Butanol-extractable iodide test, 61

Calcitonin, medullary carcinoma and, 48
Camera, gamma, 73
Cancer, of thyroid gland, differentiated, 145–148. See also *Carcinoma(s)*.
   medullary, 149
   undifferentiated, 150
Carcinoma(s), in ectopic thyroid, 9. See also *Cancer*.
   of thyroid gland, follicular, 44
      giant cell, 44, 46, 50

Carcinoma(s) (*Continued*)
   of thyroid gland, medullary, 46, *47*
      papillary, 41, *41*, *42*, *43*
      spindle cell, 50
      undifferentiated, 48, *49*, *51*
   thyroiditis and, 129
Carotid sinus syndrome, 162
Carotodynia, 55
Cell(s), Hürthle, 24
   oxyphilic, 24
Cervicomediastinotomy, *195*, *196*
Chauliac, 1
Children, antithyroid treatment in, 113
Choriocarcinoma, thyroid function and, 99
Cretinism, goitrous, 65
Crile, 3
Cyst(s), thyroglossal, 5
      infection of, 6
      treatment of, 6

de Quervain's disease, 126
de Vigo, 1
Diiodotyrosine, 56
Drugs, antithyroid, thyroid surgery and, 155
   thyroactive, 68

Edema, pretibial, Graves' disease and, 32
Exophthalmos, 32
   malignant, tests for, 67
Eye, changes in, in Graves' disease, 103, 105–107

Fistula(s), thyroglossal, 5

203

Globus hystericus, 55
Goiter, adenomatous, 27, *28, 29, 30,*
    121-125. See also *Goiter, nodular, nontoxic.*
  causes of, 27
  clinical aspects of, 122
  complications of, 30
  diagnosis of, 123
    differential, 124
  etiology of, 121
  treatment of, 124
 colloid, 28
 diffuse, 29
 diffuse toxic, 31, 65, 99-107. See also *Graves' disease.*
 endemic, 29
 exophthalmic, 31
 history of, operative, 1-4
 infrahyoid, 7
 intrathoracic, 196, *197*
 iodine-deficient, 29
 lingual, 7, *7, 8*
 mediastinal, *123*
 nodular, 28
   nontoxic, 121-125. See also *Goiter, adenomatous.*
   toxic, 107. See also *Plummer's disease.*
   tests for, 66
 removal of, 129
 substernal, freeing of, 192, *194*
 suprahyoid, 7
Graves' disease, 31, *32,* 99-107. See also *Goiter, diffuse, toxic.*
  clinical manifestations of, 101
  differential diagnosis of, 104
  etiology of, 100
  eye changes in, 103, 105-107
  myxedema and, 103
  pathogenesis of, 100
  physical findings in, 103
  recurrent, 111
  skin in, 104
  tests for, 65
Günther, 2

Halsted, 3
Hamolsky test, 83
Hashimoto's disease, 35, *36,* 127
  complications of, 36
  tests for, 66
Hemithyroidectomy, left subtotal, 188
Hemorrhage, following thyroidectomy, 198
  in thyroid surgery, 162
Hydatidiform mole, thyroid function and, 99
Hyperparathyroidism, thyroid gland and, 80

Hyperthyroidism, 99-120
  postoperative, 200
  preoperative evaluation in, 69
  primary, 31
  remission in, 114
  secondary, 30
  surgery for, emergency, anesthesia for, 166
  treatment of, 109-114
    medical, long-term, 113
    radioiodine, 111
    surgical, 110
Hypoparathyroidism, post-thyroidectomy, 200
Hypothyroidism, Hashimoto's disease and, 36
  postoperative, 200

^{123}I, 74
^{125}I, 74
^{131}I, 73
Iodine, radioactive, in thyroid gland scanning, 71, 73
  in thyroid tumors, 142
Isthmus of thyroid gland, division of, 186, *187*

Kendall, 2
Kocher, 2

Lahey, 3
Laryngeal nerve. See *Nerve(s), laryngeal.*
Liotrix, 68
Lobectomy of thyroid gland, 138, 141
Long-acting thyroid stimulator, 67
Lung, carcinoma of, metastatic, 77
Lusitanus, 1
Lymphoma of thyroid gland, 51

MacCallum, 2
MacKenzie, 4
Mandt, 2
Mayo brothers, 3
Mediastinotomy, transsternal, 195, *197*
Mediastinum, dissection of, 141
Methimazole, in hyperthyroidism, 113, 114
  toxic reactions to, 114
Monoiodotyrosine, 56
Murphy-Pattee test, 83
Muscle(s), prethyroid, division of, 174-178, *177*
  sternocleidomastoid, 11

Index

Muscle(s) (Continued)
  sternohyoid, 11
    division of, 174, *176*, *177*
  sternothyroid, 11
    division of, 174, *176*, *177*
Muys, 1
Myasthenia gravis, Graves' disease and, 102
Myxedema, 65
  Graves' disease and, 103
  permanent, radioiodine and, 112
  preoperative evaluation in, 69
  primary, vs. secondary, 82

Neck, dissection of, 141
  radical, 138
    thyroidectomy and, 189–192
      incision for, *190*, *191*, *192*, *193*
  muscles of, 10, *12*
  skin of, 10
Nerve(s), ansa hypoglossi, 11
  laryngeal, *17*, *20*, *21*
    paralysis of, 22
    recurrent, isolation of, *181*, *182*
  thyroid artery and, *19*
Neurofibromatosis, medullary carcinoma and, 48

Paralysis, hypokalemic periodic, Graves' disease and, 102
Parathyroid glands, identification of, 185, *186*
Paulus, 1
Pheochromocytoma, thyroid gland and, 80
Platysma, 10, *11*
  division of, 173, *173*
Plummer, 2
Plummer's disease, 107. See also *Goiter, nodular, toxic.*
  tests for, 66
  laboratory, 109
Pregnancy, antithyroid treatment in, 113
  radioiodine and, 111
Prethyroid muscles, division of, 174–178, *177*
Propylthiouracil, in hyperthyroidism, 113, 114
  toxic reactions to, 114
Protein-bound iodine test, 61
Psammoma bodies, 41, *43*
Pyramidal lobe, thyroid in, 7

Radioactive iodine uptake test, 63
Radioiodine, minimum effective dose, 112
  myxedema and, 112

Radionuclides for thyroid gland scanning, 73
Riedel's struma, 34, 128

Scanner, rectilinear, 72
Scanography of thyroid gland, 71
Selenomethionine-75 in thyroid gland scanning, 75
Serum, thyroid function tests on, 60
Sipple's syndrome, 48
Skin, in Graves' disease, 104
  of neck, 10
Sternohyoid muscles, 11
  division of, 174, *176*, *177*
Sternothyroid muscles, 11
  division of, 174, *176*, *177*
Struma, Hashimoto's. See *Struma lymphomatosa.*
  Riedel's, 34, 128
Struma lymphomatosa, 35, *36*, 127
  complications of, 35, 36

T3 test, 66, 83
T4 test, 83
Technetium-99 in thyroid gland scanning, 74
Thiocarbamides in hyperthyroidism, 113
Thiouracil in hyperthyroidism, 113
Thyrobinding index, 83
Thyrocalcitonin, 69
Thyroglobulin, 24
Thyroglossal cysts, 5, *6*
Thyroglossal duct, 25, *27*
  tumors of, 26
Thyroid, desiccated, 68, 114
  ectopic, 6
    carcinoma in, 9
  extract of, suppressive therapy with, 142
  lingual, 7, 25, *26*
Thyroid artery, inferior, isolation of, 180, *181*
Thyroid crisis, 115
Thyroid gland, abnormalities of, 77
  developmental, 5–9
  adenoma of, 37, *37*, *38*, 107
  anatomy of, surgical, 10–23
  blood vessels supplying, 12, *13*
  carcinoma of, differentiated, 145–148
    follicular, 44, *45*
    giant cell, 44, *46*, 50
    medullary, 46, *47*, 149
    metastasis from, 77
    papillary, 41, *41*, *42*, *43*
    secondary, 50
    spindle cell, 50
    undifferentiated, 48, *49*, *51*, 150

Thyroid gland (*Continued*)
  diseases of, 64
    quantitative, 65
  embryology of, 5-9
  enlargement of, 103
  exposure of, anterior, 171
  follicles of, 24
  formation of, disorders of, 64
  function of, assessment of, 80
    tests of, laboratory, 105
  hyperactivity of, 26
  hyperparathyroidism and, 80
  hyperplasia of, primary, 31
  inferior pole of, mobilization of, 182, *183*
  iodide excess in, 64
  iodide lack in, 64
  isthmus of, 24
    division of, 186, *187*
    resection of, 141
  lobectomy of, 138
    contralateral radical subtotal, 141
  lobes of, 24
  lymphatic vessels draining, 15, *16*
  lymphoma of, 51
  metastatic disease of, 77
  mobilization of, 178, *179*
  morphology of, 76
  nodule(s) of, abnormal function and, 134
    change in size of, 134
    clinical evaluation of, 133
    cold, 79
    diagnosis of, 135
    excision of, 139
    hoarseness and, 134
    hot, 78
    management of, 136
    pain in, 134
    physical examination of, 135
    radiation therapy and, 134
    surgery for, selection of, 140
    swallowing difficulty and, 135
  normal, 24, *25*, 76, *76*
  palpation of, *122*
  pheochromocytoma and, 80
  physiology of, 55-70, 80
  radioisotope scanning of, instrumentation for, 72
    radionuclides for, 73
    surgical significance of, 71-98
  scan of, case studies of, 84-96
  superior vessels of, division of, 183, *184*
  suppression of, test of, 82
  surgery of, anesthesia for, 153-169
      selection of, 158
    antithyroid drugs in, 155
    preoperative medication in, 157
    preoperative preparation of patient for, 155
  surgical pathology of, 24-54

Thyroid gland (*Continued*)
  tests of, functional, 55-70, *58*
    on serum, 60
    peripheral, 63
  tumors of, 133-152
    benign, 36
    chemotherapy in, 144
    irradiation in, supervoltage external, 143
    malignant, 39
      classification of, 40
    radioactive iodine in, 142
    upper pole of, mobilization of, 183, *184*, *185*
  uptake of radioactive iodine by, study of, 81
Thyroid-stimulating hormone, 26
Thyroid storm, 115
  treatment of, 115
Thyroid tissue, extracervical, 77
Thyroidectomy, closure of, 188
  complications of, management of, 161
    postoperative, 198
      pulmonary, 163
      wound, 198
  elevation of skin flap for, 173, *174*
  hemorrhage following, 198
  incision for, 171, *172*
  neck dissection and, 189-192
    incision for, *190*, *191*, *192*, *193*
  position for, *160*, 171, *171*
  postoperative position, *161*
  respiratory obstruction following, 163, 199
  subtotal, 110, 131
  technique of, 170-201
  vocal cord paralysis and, 131
Thyroiditis, 33, 126-132
  acute suppurative, 126
  autoimmune, 35
  carcinoma and, 129
  chronic, 127
    nonspecific, 33, *33*
  classification of, 126-129
  de Quervain's, 34
  diagnosis of, 129
  granulomatous, 34
  Hashimoto's. See *Hashimoto's disease.*
  invasive fibrous, 34
  lymphocytic, 35
  neck pressure symptoms in, 129
  nonspecific, 128
  pseudotuberculous, 34
  subacute, 34, *35*, 127
    tests for, 67
  surgery in, indications for, 129
  viral, 34
Thyrotoxicosis, 99-107. See also *Graves' disease.*
  factitial, 105
  T3 tests for, 66, 83
Thyrotropin-releasing hormone, 57

Thyrotropin-stimulating hormone, 57
Thyroxine, 26, 57
    action of, mechanism of, 57
    synthetic, 68
Thyroxine-binding globulin, 57
Thyroxine-binding prealbumin, 57
Thyroxine displacement test, 62
Thyroxine iodide test, 62
Thyroxine uptake test, 61
Trachea, hole in, thyroid surgery and, 162
Tracheotomy, 164, *165*
Triiodothyronine, 57
    action of, mechanism of, 57
    radioactive, 83
Triiodothyronine sodium liothyronine, 68

Tumors of thyroid gland, 133–152

Vein(s), inferior, 14
    jugular, 12
    thyroid, deep, 13
        lateral, 14
        superficial, 12
        superior, 14
Vocal cord, paralysis of, thyroidectomy and, 131
Voegtlin, 2
von Eiselsberg, 2
von Walther, 1